Emergency Department Critical Care

Edited by

Donald M. Yealy, MD

Professor and Chair
Department of Emergency Medicine; and
Professor of Medicine, and Clinical and Translational Sciences
University of Pittsburgh
Pittsburgh, PA

Clifton W. Callaway, MD, PhD

Professor and Executive Vice Chair
Department of Emergency Medicine
University of Pittsburgh
Pittsburgh, Pennsylvania

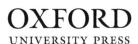

OXFORD
UNIVERSITY PRESS

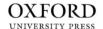

OXFORD

UNIVERSITY PRESS

Oxford University Press is a department of the University of
Oxford. It furthers the University's objective of excellence
in research, scholarship, and education by publishing worldwide.

Oxford   New York
Auckland   Cape Town   Dar es Salaam   Hong Kong   Karachi
Kuala Lumpur   Madrid   Melbourne   Mexico City   Nairobi
New Delhi   Shanghai   Taipei   Toronto

With offices in
Argentina   Austria   Brazil   Chile   Czech Republic   France   Greece
Guatemala   Hungary   Italy   Japan   Poland   Portugal   Singapore
South Korea   Switzerland   Thailand   Turkey   Ukraine   Vietnam

Oxford is a registered trade mark of Oxford University Press in the UK and certain other
countries.

Published in the United States of America by
Oxford University Press
198 Madison Avenue, New York, NY 10016

© Oxford University Press 2013

Library of Congress Cataloging-in-Publication Data
   Emergency department critical care / edited by Donald M. Yealy, Clifton W. Callaway.
   p. ; cm.—(Pittsburgh critical care medicine series)
   Includes bibliographical references and index.
   ISBN 978-0-19-977912-3 (alk. paper)—ISBN 978-0-19-997635-5
   (alk. paper)—ISBN 978-0-19-997636-2 (alk. paper)
   I. Yealy, Donald M.   II. Callaway, Clifton W.   III. Series: Pittsburgh critical care medicine.
   [DNLM: 1. Critical Care—methods.   2. Critical Illness—therapy.   3. Emergency
   Service, Hospital.   4. Emergency Treatment—methods. WX 218]
   LC Classification not assigned
   616.02'8—dc23
   2012039791

9 8 7 6 5 4 3 2 1
Printed in the United States of America
on acid-free paper

Series Preface

No place in the world is more closely identified with critical care medicine than Pittsburgh. In the late 1960s, Peter Safar and Ake Grenvik pioneered the science and practice of critical care not just in Pittsburgh but around the world. Their multidisciplinary team approach became the standard for how ICU care is delivered in Pittsburgh to this day. The Pittsburgh Critical Care Medicine series honors this tradition. Edited and largely authored by University of Pittsburgh faculty, the content reflects best practice in critical care medicine. The Pittsburgh model has been adopted by many programs around the world, and local leaders are recognized as world leaders. It is our hope that through this series of concise handbooks a small part of this tradition can be passed on to the many practitioners of critical care the world over.

John A. Kellum
Series Editor

>

Contents

Part II: Methodology and Procedures

Preface

The care of those with critical illness is best started early to avoid the cascade of adaptive and maladaptive events that can worsen outcomes. In this text, we seek to identify the presentations of selected critical illnesses in the emergency department (ED) and to guide the bedside provider. We target common categories of acute illness and describe the use of key approaches to assess illness and improve care. Each chapter is meant to stand alone and provide practical advice.

We recognize that some critical events and illnesses are not covered here, and in-depth discussion of other topics can be found in companion texts in this series. Our goal is to focus on the ED needs and to deliver pragmatic advice to guide common needs, complementing the care before and after this interval. This approach has been central here at the University of Pittsburgh based on the efforts of early thought leaders including Peter Safar and Ronald Stewart. These pioneers saw the value of early care, starting at first patient contact and merging with later efforts. We eschew a detailed analysis of all potential mechanisms and therapies and instead seek concise readability.

We thank the series editor for recognizing this important niche, and we hope that our readers will deliver better care because of the insight from the authors.

Donald M. Yealy, MD
Clifton W. Callaway, MD, PhD

Acknowledgments

We thank the authors and the publishing staff for their effort, diligence, knowledge, and patience. Just as important are our partners, who created and sustained a milieu of excellence in emergency and critical care.

Finally, we thank our wives and families, who supported us as we dedicated time to this text and to emergency care.

DMY
CWC

Contributors

Opeolu Adeoye, MD

Assistant Professor of Emergency
Medicine and Neurosurgery
University of Cincinnati
Cincinnati, OH

John H. Burton, MD

Professor of Emergency Medicine
Virginia Tech Carilion School of
Medicine
Chair, Department of Emergency
Medicine
Carilion Clinic
Virginia Tech Carilion School
of Medicine
Roanoke, VA

Clifton W. Callaway, MD, PhD

Professor and Executive Vice Chair
Department of Emergency Medicine
University of Pittsburgh
Pittsburgh, PA

Jestin N. Carlson, MD

Clinical Assistant Professor
of Emergency Medicine
University of Pittsburgh
Pittsburgh, PA

Lillian Emlet, MD

Assistant Professor of Critical
Care and Emergency Medicine
University of Pittsburgh
Pittsburgh, PA

Raquel Forsythe, MD

Assistant Professor of Surgery and
Critical Care Medicine
University of Pittsburgh
Pittsburgh, PA

David F. Gaieski, MD

Associate Professor
Department of Emergency Medicine
University of Pennsylvania Perleman
School of Medicine
and
Clinical Director
Center for Resuscitation Science
Philadelphia, PA

Munish Goyal, MD

Associate Professor of Emergency
Medicine
Georgetown University
and
Director, Emergency Critical Care
MedStar Washington Hospital Center
Washington, DC

Alan C. Heffner, MD

Director, Medical Intensive Care Unit
Pulmonary and Critical Care
Consultants
Department of Internal Medicine
Department of Emergency Medicine
Carolinas Medical Center
and
Assistant Clinical Professor
University of North Carolina School
of Medicine
Charlotte, NC

J. Stephen Huff, MD

Associate Professor, Emergency
Medicine and Neurology
Department of Emergency Medicine
University of Virginia Health Sciences
Center
Charlottesville, Virginia

Robert J. Hyde, MD

Assistant Director of Ultrasound,
Department of Emergency Medicine
Dartmouth Hitchcock Medical
Center
Lebanon, NH

Edward C. Jauch, MD

Professor, Division of Emergency
Medicine, Department of Medicine,
and
Department of Neurosciences
Medical University of South Carolina
Charleston, SC

Alan E. Jones, MD

Professor of Emergency Medicine
Department of Emergency Medicine
University of Mississippi Medical Center
Jackson, MS

John A. Kellum, MD

Professor and Vice-Chair
Department of Critical Care
Medicine
University of Pittsburgh
Pittsburgh, PA

Khoshal Latifzai, MD

Department of Emergency Medicine
Yale School of Medicine
New Haven, CT

Eric J. Lavonas, MD

Associate Director
Rocky Mountain Poison and Drug
Center
Denver Health and Hospital
Authority
Denver, Colorado
and
Associate Professor
Department of Emergency Medicine
University of Colorado School of
Medicine
Aurora, Colorado

Glen E. Michael, MD

Department of Emergency Medicine
University of Virginia
Charlottesville, VA

H. Bryant Nguyen, MD, MS

Director, Emergency Critical Care
Associate Professor
Department of Emergency Medicine
and
Department of Medicine, Critical
Care
Loma Linda University

**Robert E. O'Connor,
MD, MPH**

Professor and Chair
Department of Emergency
Medicine
University of Virginia School of
Medicine
Charlottesville, VA

William Frank Peacock, MD

Professor and Vice Chair of
Emergency Medicine
Baylor University
Houston, TX

Edward P. Sloan, MD, MPH

Professor
Department of Emergency
Medicine
University of Illinois at Chicago
Chicago, IL

Robert D. Stevens, MD

Associate Professor of
Anesthesiology Critical Care
Medicine, Neurology, Neurosurgery,
and Radiology
Johns Hopkins University School
of Medicine
Baltimore, MD

Stephen Trzeciak, MD, MPH
Associate Professor
Departments of Medicine and
Emergency Medicine
Cooper Medical School of Rowan
University
Camden, NJ

Tertius Tuy, MD
Changi General Hospital Singapore,
Singapore

Henry E. Wang, MD, MS
Associate Professor of Emergency
Medicine
University of Alabama - Birmingham
Birmingham, AL

Charles R. Wira III, MD
Assistant Professor
Department of Emergency Medicine
Yale School of Medicine
New Haven, CT

Donald M. Yealy, MD
Professor and Chair
Department of Emergency Medicine
and
Professor of Medicine, and Clinical
and Translational Sciences
University of Pittsburgh
Pittsburgh, PA

Part I

Clinical Syndromes

Chapter 1

Approach to Undifferentiated Organ Failure/Shock ("Blue or Bad")

Lillian Emlet

Introduction

Systemic blood pressure is a by-product of cardiac output combined with systemic vascular resistance. Hypotension is often defined as systolic blood pressure (SBP) <100 mmHg or mean arterial pressure (MAP) <65 mmHg, but in practice this or any cutoff value is arbitrary, since end-organ hypoperfusion or organ dysfunction and clinically relevant shock can be present despite a "normal SBP." Thus, while "hypotension" is shock, all shock is not hypotensive in presentation.

Traditional classifications of shock include distributive shock, cardiogenic shock, hypovolemic shock, and obstructive shock. Physical exam findings and measured blood laboratory values guide the resuscitation and titration of inotropes, vasopressors, volume expanders, and mechanical assist devices. A systematic approach to undifferentiated hypotension allows a stepwise method to resuscitate and diagnose the etiology of shock, as there may be multiple processes occurring simultaneously.

Clinically relevant shock states are a result of tissue hypoperfusion and tissue oxygen transport. Below threshold tissue oxygen content, a decrease in ventilatory oxygen consumption (VO_2) causes inadequate energy delivery and increased lactic acid production. Decreases in oxygen delivery can be from hypoxia, anemia, cardiac failure, or increased demand. Detecting shock and resuscitation adequacy can be done via physical exam, measurements of oxygen delivery (central venous or mixed venous saturation), and measurements of tissue perfusion (lactate, base deficit, or gastric tonometry).

Definition of Terms

Afterload: the pressure that the ventricle must overcome to eject blood volume, determined by size and thickness of ventricle, vascular tone, and volume of blood

Cardiac index (CI): CO/body surface area (BSA)—2.5–4 L/min per M^2

Cardiac output (CO): volume of blood ejected by ventricle in 1 minute, 4–8 L/min, heart rate multiplied by stroke volume

Cardiogenic shock (CS): primary cardiac pump failure resulting in decreased end-organ perfusion

Central venous pressure (CVP): venous pressure measured at the right atrium; normal is 8–12 mm Hg, but what is key is not the absolute measurement but the response to therapy

Diastolic blood pressure (DBP): pressure of blood at the end of the left ventricular filling in late diastole

Distributive shock: inadequate end-organ perfusion from decreased systemic vascular resistance and high CO; also known as vasodilatory shock

Hypotension: systolic blood pressure <90 mm Hg, MAP <65 mm Hg, relative drop in baseline SBP >40–50 mm Hg; clinically significant hypotension entails signs and symptoms of decreased end-organ perfusion

Hypovolemic shock: decreased intravascular volume resulting in adequate end-organ perfusion

Mean arterial pressure (MAP): (SBP + 2×DBP)/3

Preload: amount of volume at end of diastole in right ventricle

$ScvO_2$: central venous oxygen saturation measured from SVC outside RA

Shock index: heart rate divided by the systolic blood pressure (HR/SBP) with normal values ranging from 0.5 to 0.7

Stroke volume (SV): difference in blood volume in ventricle between end diastole and end systole; three determinants of SV are preload, afterload, and contractility; normal value is 60–100 mL

SvO_2: true mixed venous oxygen saturation measured from pulmonary artery (Swan-Ganz) catheter

Systemic vascular resistance (SVR): resistance to blood flow from peripheral vasculature

Systolic blood pressure (SBP): pressure of blood at the end of the stroke output of left ventricle

Clinical Syndromes (Symptom and Organ Based)

General findings of shock can vary, and they can be subtle in some patients. These include the following:

Cardiovascular: myocardial ischemia and infarction

Gastrointestinal: abdominal pain out of proportion, gastrointestinal bleeding, and necrosis

Neurologic: altered mental status, including confusion, somnolence, encephalopathy, and coma

Pulmonary: respiratory insufficiency (bradypnea, tachypnea), increased work of breathing (accessory muscle use, sternocleidomastoid muscle use, abdominal breathing, diaphoresis, nasal flaring), respiratory arrest/failure, hypoxia via atelectasis, and compensatory shunting

Renal: decreased urine output

Skin: mottling; decreased capillary refill; decreased turgor; warm, dry skin; warm, clammy skin; diaphoresis; cool skin; cyanosis; livedo reticularis

Physical exam findings can be misleading, and more than one mechanism of shock can exist simultaneously.

Distributive shock has many underlying causes: adrenal insufficiency, anaphylactic shock, decompensated liver failure, thyrotoxicosis, medication side effects (vasodilatory drugs), septic shock, neurogenic spinal shock, and sympatholytic effects of high thoracic epidural. The classic physical exam findings are warm, flushed skin; pitting edema; tachycardia; or tachypnea (early compensation), though commonly one or more are missing.

Hypovolemic shock can present from hemorrhage (retroperitoneal, gastrointestinal, intraabdominal, trauma, surgical sites), gastrointestinal losses (vomiting and diarrhea), renal losses (excessive diuresis, diabetes insipidus), and third-spacing processes (severe protein-deficient malnutrition, large third-degree burns, severe pancreatitis, cirrhosis, congestive heart failure, nephrotic syndrome, sepsis-mediated capillary leak into extravascular space). The classic physical exam findings are pale skin with decreased capillary refill, cool skin with decreased turgor, or decreased urine output.

Cardiogenic shock results from right heart failure, left heart failure (myocardial infarction, ventricular wall rupture), arrhythmias (atrial fibrillation/flutter with rapid ventricular response, supraventricular tachycardias, complete heart block, junctional rhythms, sinus bradycardia, second-degree heart block type 2, ventricular tachycardia), and severe valvular disease (critical aortic stenosis, aortic insufficiency, mitral regurgitation, mitral stenosis). The classic physical exam findings are cool extremities with decreased capillary refill, mottling, or decreased urine output.

Obstructive shock can emanate from tension pneumothorax, cardiac tamponade, or large pulmonary emboli. The classic physical exam findings are cool extremities, decreased capillary refill, mottling, distended neck veins, or muffled heart or lung sounds.

General and Key Management Controversies

Assessing oxygenation and ventilation is the key first step in shock patients, and this is addressed in Chapter 3.

Adequate Fluid Resuscitation

Treatment and monitoring of resuscitation occurs simultaneously through bedside observations, using both invasive and noninvasive tools, and serial laboratory testing. *Traditional physical exam findings* involve measuring vital signs and examination of skin perfusion, neurologic status, and urine output, but these *can easily fail to identify successful or inadequate resuscitation*.

Because of this, invasive measurements of central venous pressure (CVP) via a central line and continuous arterial blood pressure via an arterial line allow for a more rapid method to measure adequacy of fluid resuscitation. *Fluid responsiveness is more important than the absolute CVP value* to help determine whether continued fluid boluses are necessary. Only half of patients with shock are fluid responsive. Choice of fluid (colloid, crystalloid, blood) and volume expanders matters less than the need to administer adequate amounts of fluid. Fluid should be given only while patient shows a response (blood pressure, CVP, clinical features); more boluses after this may cause right ventricular overload and decreased cardiac output. Another simple test is to raise the legs 30 degrees in a supine patient with an arterial line in place; an increased blood pressure transiently or an increase in pulse amplitude changes (pulse pressure) means more fluid may help.

Laboratory values that can be measured serially to assess adequacy of resuscitation include $ScvO_2$, lactate, and base deficit. A common $ScvO_2$ target is 70% or greater (correlating to a true SvO_2 of 75%) after ensuring the CVP is normalized. Lactate clearance, defined as a drop to normal or at least 10% every 1–2 hours, is another method of ensuring adequate resuscitation.

A variety of invasive and noninvasive devices may aid in assessing adequacy of fluid resuscitation or vasoactive drug use, from a pulmonary artery catheter to noninvasive Doppler measurements of cardiac output and tissue oxygenation. In sedated, intubated, and ventilated patients, measurements of systolic pressure variation (SPV), pulse pressure variation, and stroke volume variation (SVV) are used in flow-monitoring devices (i.e., Edwards FloTrac, Pulsion LiCCO, LiDCO Group LiDCO). Preload dependency occurs until SPV is <10 mm Hg, SVV is <10%, and change in pulse pressure variation is <13%. These methods are inaccurate in patients who are spontaneously breathing or have arrhythmias. These methods are also inaccurate if catheter-derived waveforms are of poor quality. These topics are covered in greater detail in Chapter 14.

Vasopressor Choice

Vasopressors affect vascular tone and cardiac contractility (inotropy) to support MAP and tissue perfusion. Catecholamines vary in the amount of inotropy, chronotropy (heart rate), vasodilation, and vasoconstriction. *There is no one vasopressor that is preferred over another*; instead types of shock states determine the utility of which agent or combinations will be most useful.

In vasodilatory shock from sepsis, most commonly used agents are norepinephrine or dopamine due to the ability to work as a peripheral vasoconstrictor via alpha 1 receptors in medium arterioles. Due to the negative inotropic effects of severe septic shock, both agents are favored due to their beta-agonist and positive chronotropic effects, therefore positively affecting cardiac output. Second-line agents include vasopressin and epinephrine, both best administered after adequate fluid resuscitation due to potent vasoconstricting properties.

Table 1.1 Properties of Vasoactive Drug Infusions

Vasopressor	Dosage	β1	β2	α1	Effects
Dopamine	5–20 mcg/kg per minute	++	+	++	↑CI ↑MAP ↑SVR
Dobutamine	2.5–20 mcg/kg per minute	+++	+	+	↑CI
Norepinephrine	0.04–1 mcg/kg per minute	++	–	+++	↑MAP ↑SVR
Phenylephrine	0.5–5 mcg/kg per minute	–	–	+++	↑MAP ↑SVR
Epinephrine	0.05–2 mcg/kg per minute	+++	++	+++	↑CI ↑MAP ↑SVR
Vasopressin	0.04 U/min	–	–	+++	↑MAP ↑SVR
Milrinone	0.375–0.75 mcg/kg per minute	(++)	–	(+)	↑CI

An advantage of epinephrine includes inotropic support, whereas advantages of vasopression include the repletion of relative lack of endogenous pituitary hormone and pure alpha constriction.

In pure cardiogenic shock, more than one agent or a mechanical device may be needed to increase the inotropic contractility of a failing ventricle and simultaneously reduce afterload. First-choice inotropes include dobutamine and dopamine, with dobutamine preferred because of afterload reduction (see Table 1.1). Both can cause tachycardia via their activation of cardiac beta receptors, which can be counterproductive in severe cardiomyopathy. An alternative is milrinone, which is metabolized via cyclic GMP in cardiac myocytes and provides inotropic support and afterload reduction with a lesser degree of tachycardia side effect than dobutamine or dopamine.

For the most severe cardiogenic shock, mechanical afterload reduction with an intraaortic balloon pump is important to consider early prior to worsening multiorgan failure (i.e., shock liver, acute renal failure). For the most severe cases of cardiac failure, extracorporeal membrane oxygenation (ECMO), left ventricular assist devices (LVADs), right ventricular assist devices (RVADs), or biventricular assist devices (BiVADs) may need to be considered. Serial transthoracic or transesophageal echocardiography is important to assess contractility and wall motion.

Methods of Assessing Resuscitative Efforts

Aside from the previously described continuous monitoring by oximetric ScvO$_2$ catheters, Swan-Ganz pulmonary artery catheters, and arterial pulse-pressure variation, noninvasive techniques include esophageal Doppler, LiDCO, and point-of-care echocardiography. Of particular utility is the use of echocardiography, since causes such as large pulmonary emboli, cardiac tamponade, and ventricular free wall rupture can be detected. Additionally, ventricular, valvular, and regional wall motion abnormalities can be assessed. Ultrasound can also diagnose pneumothorax, IVC size, and volume/preload status dynamically over time. As noted earlier, *using CVP alone outside of extreme values is not prudent* without additional information for fluid responsiveness since there is a poor correlation between CVP and preload.

Optimally, serial and multimodal attempts to assess adequacy of resuscitation are necessary. Watching physiologic exam findings (urine output, skin examination, neurologic awakening) combined with objective laboratory measurements (lactate, ScvO$_2$) over short periods (1–2 hours) of aliquots of titrated treatment (fluid bolus, blood transfusion, addition of inotrope) provides the best method to monitor resuscitation. *Using a combination of methods allows for a more global assessment of perfusion* since no single method is a gold standard of measurement.

Weaning and Titrating Vasopressors

After initiation of vasopressors and inotropes, titration remains an ongoing process of looking at both absolute values (i.e., CVP, MAP, lactate) and physical exam findings (e.g., shock index, urine output). First, adequate preload restoration via fluid and blood to treat hypovolemia is necessary, and any hemorrhage needs to be controlled. In distributive shock, the new volume of distribution can be quite large and requires generous amounts of fluids; there is a balance, since overzealous volume can increase mortality. Again, a multimodal close assessment can be a useful method to watch closely (i.e., hourly) the responses in distributive shock. Even with low cardiac ejection fractions, correction to adequate preload is important in cardiogenic shock, and the subsequent titration off of vasoactive agents is made in slower blocks of time (i.e., over 6–12 hours).

Generally, catechol vasopressors (norepinephrine, neosynephrine) can be titrated quickly. Inotropes (milrinone, dopamine, dobutamine, epinephrine) are titrated less quickly (every few hours) ideally with definable cardiac endpoints (ScvO$_2$, CO, or CI). Vasopressin, is initiated at a fixed dose for catecholamine-refractory shock, and is discontinued after weaning of catechol vasopressors to modest levels. Parameters for titration, usually MAP 60–70, for vasopressors should be explicit and timed (e.g., every 2–4 hours).

Transitioning to the Intensive Care Unit

Aside from measurement of blood pressure and physiologic endpoints, as mentioned earlier, ensuring complete assessment and treatment in preparation for ongoing care allows a smoother transition to the intensive care unit (ICU). Depending on length of time in the emergency department (ED), serial assessments may be necessary for both nurses and physicians. Optimally, every 2 hours, assessments of sedation, urine output, and vitals are made. Every 4 hours, repeat laboratories should be checked as the clinical situation warrants, notably lactate, $ScvO_2$, ABG or venous gas, and hemoglobin. Protocol checklists for ED nurses allow physicians to clarify these tasks. In most patients, keeping the head of the bed at 30 degrees will help prevent aspiration.

Respiratory therapists should also report abnormalities every 4 hours to make appropriate ventilator changes. For extended ICU care provided in ED-based critical care units, local ICU protocols should be implemented in terms of frequency of specialized examinations (e.g., neurologic and vascular exams), laboratories, prophylactic care (e.g., stress ulcer prophylaxis, DVT prophylaxis), antibiotics, and other therapeutic agents.

Communication with family regarding goals of therapy and prognosis can be initiated in the ED. Despite barriers to communication such as difficulty in locating family members or finding a quiet location for disclosure of bad news, the discussion of goals of therapy, bad news, prognosis, and expectations for symptom management can be achieved. Attention to communicating expectations for symptom management, prognosis, and transition of care from the ED to the ICU helps provide families with seamless care; attention to communicating resuscitative endpoints to the ICU team helps provide seamless resuscitation.

Summary to the Initial Emergency Department Resuscitation Approach

- Do an early airway assessment and use oxygen liberally.
- Obtain adequate intravenous (IV) access (two large-bore 16-gauge IVs, introducer, or central line; internal jugular preferred over subclavian or femoral).
- Obtain appropriate laboratories (complete blood count [CBC] with differential, basic metabolic panel [BMP], coagulation profile [PT/INR/PTT], type and screen, lactate, arterial or venous blood gas [ABG or VBG], and liver function tests [LFT])
- Fluid bolus 500–1000 mL lactated ringers or saline while determining shock etiologies.
- Consider ultrasound to assess cardiac function, IVC size and filling, and to detect intra-abdominal hemorrhage (eFAST or RUSH exam).
- Reassess endpoints of resuscitation every hour with more than one endpoint (such as lactate or ScvO2), starting with vital signs and physical exam.

Pearls of Care

1. Early fluid boluses while initiating attempts for invasive (central venous catheter and arterial catheter) and noninvasive monitoring (point-of-care ultrasound and echocardiography) are best to optimize success of resuscitation.
2. Frequent and multimodal serial assessment of adequacy of resuscitation is essential (i.e., serum lactate, urine output, central venous pressure, response to fluid challenge, physical exam).

3. Ensure adequate volume repletion prior to initiation of second-line vasopressors.
4. In cases of continued severe shock despite adequate volume repletion, correction of metabolic acidosis, and vasopressor/inotrope initiation, consider cardiac tamponade, ventricular (right or left) heart failure, and relative adrenal insufficiency.
5. More than one shock state can coexist (i.e., distributive and cardiogenic) and require simultaneous treatments and monitoring.

Selected Readings

Arnold RC, Shapiro NI, Jones AE, et al. Multicenter study of early lactate clearance as a determinant of survival in patients with presumed sepsis. *Shock* 2009;32:35–39.

Dellinger RP, Levy MM, Carlet JM, et al. Surviving Sepsis Campaign: international guidelines for management of severe sepsis and septic shock: 2008. *Crit Care Med* 2008; 36: 1394–1396.

Emanuel LL, Quest TE, eds. *The EPEC Project. The Education in Palliative and End-of-life Care for Emergency Medicine (EPEC-TM) Curriculum*. Chicago, IL: Northwestern University, 2008.

Jones AE, Shapiro NI, Trzeciak S, et al. Lactate clearance vs. central venous oxygen saturation as goals of early sepsis therapy: a randomized clinical trial. *JAMA* 2010;303(8):739–746.

Jones AE, Tayal VS, Sullivan M, Kline JA. Randomized controlled trial of immediate versus delayed goal-directed ultrasound to identify the cause of nontraumatic hypotension in emergency department patients. *Crit Care Med* 2004;32:1703–1708.

Marik PE, Baram M, Vahid B. Does central venous pressure predict fluid responsiveness? A systematic review of the literature and the tale of seven mares. *Chest* 2008;134:172–178.

Marik PE, Cavallazzi R, Vasu T, Hirani A. Dynamic changes in arterial waveform derived variables and fluid responsiveness in mechanically ventilated patients: a systematic review of the literature. *Crit Care Med* 2009;37:2642–2647.

Marino PL, Sutin KM. *The ICU Book*. 3rd ed. Philadelphia, PA: Lippincott Williams & Wilkins; 2006.

McGee WT, Headley J, Frazier JA, eds. *Quick Guide to Cardiopulmonary Care*. 2nd ed. Edwards Lifesciences: Irvine, CA: 2010.

Perera P, Mailhot T, Riley D, Mandavia D. The RUSH exam: rapid ultrasound in shock in the evaluation of the critically ill. *Emerg Med Clin N Am* 2010;28:29–56.

Chapter 2

Sepsis and Shock with Infection

Alan E. Jones and Alan C. Heffner

Introduction

Sepsis is the tenth leading cause of death in the United States and results in an estimated 750,000 hospitalizations annually. At least one-half of these patients are admitted via the emergency department (ED), which highlights the importance of emergency care in acute sepsis management. Most concerning, sepsis carries a hospital mortality of 20%–50%.

Definition of Terms

Bacteremia: is the presence of live bacteria in the blood but exists in less than half of severe sepsis cases. In some settings, manifestations of infection arise from cytopathic or exotoxin effects in the absence of microbial tissue invasion (e.g., *C. difficile* colitis, staphylococcal toxic shock syndrome).

Systemic inflammatory response syndrome (SIRS): is the global manifestation of innate immune activation. SIRS is a generalized physiological response that is not specific to infection. The systemic immune response may be incited by diverse insults, including tissue injury (e.g., burns and trauma) and sterile inflammatory and immuno-stimulating diseases.

Sepsis syndromes: are a continuum of disease from *sepsis* (infection with inflammatory response) to *severe sepsis* (sepsis plus acute organ dysfunction) and *septic shock* (sepsis with cardiovascular failure; see Table 2.1.) Those who arrive with evidence of severe disease have an even higher morbidity and mortality, but any form of sepsis retains risk of a poor outcome.

Presenting Signs and Symptoms

Outside of extreme cases, there is no pathognomonic sign or single reliable test to diagnose early sepsis. Although the current diagnosis of sepsis is based on physiologic indicators of SIRS in the setting of infection, the clinical presentation

Table 2.1 The Sepsis Syndromes

Infection	Microbial invasion of normally sterile host tissue or fluid.
SIRS	The systemic inflammatory response to a variety of insults
	Manifested by two or more of the following:
	1) Temperature >38°C (100.4°F) or <36°C (96.8°F)
	2) Heart rate >90 beats/minute
	3) Respiratory rate >20 breaths/min or $PaCO_2$ <32 mm Hg
	4) White blood cell count >12,000/mm^3 or <4000/mm^3, or >10% immature bands
Sepsis	The systemic inflammatory response to infection
Severe sepsis	Sepsis with acute organ dysfunction:
	Acute lung injury: PaO_2/ FiO_2 <300
	Acute respiratory failure
	Acute kidney injury: Serum creatinine >0.5 mg/dL from baseline
Oliguria: UOP	<0.5 cc/kg/hr for 2 consecutive hours
	Encephalopathy ranging from confusion, apathy, or agitation
	Coagulopathy: Protime (PT) >16 seconds or a PTT >60 seconds
	Thrombocytopenia: platelet count <100,000/μL
	Hyperbilirubinemia: Serum bilirubin >4 mg/dL
	Blood lactate ≥ 4 mmol/L
	Clinical malperfusion: cool extremities, mottling, delayed capillary refill
Septic shock	Sepsis with hypotension refractory to initial fluid resuscitation (20 cc/kg)
	SBP <90 mm Hg or >40 mm Hg drop from baseline
	MAP <65 mm Hg or >25 mm Hg drop from baseline

and course of infected patients are rarely as distinct as the definitions suggest. However, *the absence of SIRS signs does not exclude clinically important infection*, as one-quarter of patients with severe sepsis do not manifest two SIRS signs at presentation. Two criteria considered classic for infection, fever and peripheral leukocytosis (with or without bandemia), are inconsistent and do not discriminate infectious from noninfectious disease. Immunocompromised and elderly patients, who are at greatest risk for severe infection, exhibit an attenuated host response, which often limits bedside detection. Difficult clinical recognition is compounded by the absence of an ideal laboratory marker(s) for sepsis.

Patients must be treated based on suspected or presumed infection. Ill-appearing patients and those presenting with unexplained SIRS or shock warrant consideration of and treatment for presumed infection.

Specific sources are more commonly associated with sepsis. Pulmonary and intra-abdominal infections account for half of severe sepsis cases. Other common high-risk sources include the urinary tract, skin and soft tissues, and endovascular sites. However, any source or agent, including atypical organisms (e.g., virus, spirochete, rickettsia, and yeast) can evolve life-threatening disease. The difficulty in clinical identification of sepsis is underscored by the fact that a primary source and site of infection remains unidentified in up to 30% of cases.

Organs Involved in Severe Sepsis and Septic Shock

Acute lung and kidney injury are the most common organ dysfunctions followed by cardiovascular, hematologic, and neurologic dysfunction. Confused, apathetic, or agitated delirium during acute sepsis is common but underappreciated. Thrombocytopenia, coagulopathy, hyperbilirubinemia, and elevated lactate are evidence of end-organ dysfunction. Mild elevations of serum creatinine (>0.5 mg/dL from baseline), even in the absence of oliguria, represent *acute kidney injury* and confer an increased risk of adverse outcome. Increasing severity of kidney dysfunction is associated with stepwise increase in mortality. Similarly, there is an additive effect of end-organ dysfunction on mortality such that three or more failing organs is associated with mortality over 60%.

Shock is a state of inadequate tissue perfusion where oxygen delivery does not meet the metabolic needs of vital tissues. Contrary to popular belief, hypotension is not a mandatory component of shock. Blood pressure is an unreliable gauge of cardiac output and oxygen delivery. Accordingly, hypoperfusion may occur with low, normal, or elevated blood pressure. *Up to half of patients with severe sepsis present in compensated shock with a normal blood pressure.* The difficulty in identifying these patients has spawned the terms *occult or cryptic shock. Uncompensated shock,* characterized by hypotension, is a late stage when attempts to maintain normal perfusion pressure are overwhelmed or exhausted. Although some patients manifest low blood pressure without apparent distress or hypoperfusion, hypotension is pathologic in the setting of acute infection. A mean arterial pressure (MAP) less than 65 mm Hg or systolic blood pressure (SBP) less than 90 mm Hg is a common threshold to define hypotension.

Transient hypotension often heralds later hemodynamic deterioration. *Transient hypotension should not be dismissed as spurious* or inconsequential.[1]

Sepsis Biomarkers

Lactate is a useful biomarker to confirm and stratify critical illness and shock. Hyperlactatemia is well recognized in the setting of acute infection and is attributed to anaerobic metabolism as a consequence of tissue hypoxia and hypoperfusion.

Blood lactate stratifies patients independent of hemodynamics and organ dysfunction.[2] Even mildly elevated (2–4 mmol/L) lactate levels are associated with increased disease severity and mortality. Among patients with suspected infection, lactate greater than 4 mmol/L is associated with a 25% death rate, 10-fold higher than patients with a normal lactate.[2] This mortality figure holds true even among patients with normal blood pressure. Arterial, venous, and capillary lactate levels are clinically equivalent and unaffected by Ringer's lactate infusion or tourniquet use.

Key Treatments

Early recognition of severe sepsis is critical and must be coupled with timely and effective therapy to improve outcome. The presence of shock, hyperlactatemia (>4 mmol/L), and/or acute organ dysfunction defines a high-risk patient group. Acute aggressive management of these patients confers short-term and persistent mortality advantage.[3]

The Institute for Healthcare Improvement and the Surviving Sepsis Campaign advocate a structured early resuscitation bundle to improve process and outcomes of patients with severe sepsis (Table 2.2). Bundle compliance generally improves with time and is associated with survival improvement.

Early Endpoint ("Goal") Directed Resuscitation

There is no single cardiovascular lesion of sepsis. Rather, sepsis and septic shock may present with a complex and dynamic cascade of cardiovascular dysfunction that includes components of hypovolemia, vasoplegia, and primary cardiac dysfunction. *Early treatment—before the cascade is profound—has the most substantial impact on outcome.* The window to reverse critical organ hypoperfusion is measured in hours starting in the ED.

Table 2.2 Treatment Components of the Surviving Sepsis Campaign Severe Sepsis Bundle
1. Measure serum lactate
2. Obtain blood cultures prior to antibiotic administration
3. Administer broad-spectrum antibiotic, within 3 hours of emergency department admission and within 1 hour of non–emergency department admission
4. In the event of hypotension and/or a serum lactate >4 mmol/L
a. Deliver an initial minimum of 20 mL/kg of crystalloid or an equivalent
b. Apply vasopressors for hypotension not responding to initial fluid resuscitation to maintain mean arterial pressure (MAP) >65 mm Hg
5. In the event of persistent hypotension despite fluid resuscitation (septic shock) and/or lactate >4 mmol/L
a. Achieve a central venous pressure (CVP) of >8 mm Hg
b. Achieve a central venous oxygen saturation ($ScvO_2$) >70% or mixed venous oxygen saturation (SvO_2) >65 %

Table 2.3 Prioritized Endpoints of Resuscitation

1) Adequate intravenous access
2) Preload optimization
a. Serial fluid challenges guided by clinical exam and patient response
b. Central venous pressure ≥8 mm Hg (≥12 mm Hg if mechanically ventilated)
c. Fluid guided by evidence of volume responsiveness gauged by dynamic hemodynamic variables
3) Mean arterial pressure (MAP) ≥65 mm Hg
4) Sustain organ perfusion and match oxygen delivery and consumption
a. Clinical regional markers
• Cutaneous perfusion
• UOP >0.5 cc/kg per hour
• Mental status
b. Global markers
• $ScvO_2$ ≥70%
• Lactate clearance (>10%)

The immediate goal of cardiovascular support is to restore and maintain systemic oxygen delivery and organ perfusion. The hemodynamic approach to patients with severe sepsis is similar to the support of other critical illness. A systematic, quantitative, goal-oriented strategy aims to rapidly optimize preload, maintain systemic perfusion pressure, and balance oxygen delivery and perfusion to meet metabolic needs (see Table 2.3).

Fluid Therapy

Initial volume expansion is achieved through rapid fluid administration under direct observation at the bedside. Crystalloid (10–20 cc/kg or 500–1000 cc) boluses should be infused over 15–30 minutes, with sequential boluses titrated to perfusion endpoints while monitoring for adverse effects, including pulmonary congestion. Colloid boluses are an option but confer no added benefit. Although total volume requirements are difficult to predict at the onset of resuscitation, empiric crystalloid loading of 50–60 cc/kg or more is common and well tolerated.

The primary goal of fluid therapy is stroke volume augmentation. Unfortunately, fluid administration does not always achieve the goal of optimizing stroke volume. Hemodynamic monitoring guides fluid management by predicting response to therapy prior to administration in hopes of avoiding ineffective and potentially deleterious fluid. Central venous pressure (CVP) is a widely advocated preload measure, but absolute values are easily misleading.

Otherwise, there is no consistent threshold of CVP to reliably define resuscitation adequacy in all patients; the responsiveness of CVP and overall clinical condition to therapy is more important than any absolute number (outside extreme values—i.e., 2 or 22 mm Hg clearly note profound fluid under- or overresuscitation). As an initial target, seek a CVP of ≥8 mm Hg in spontaneously breathing patients and ≥12 mm Hg in mechanically ventilated patients.

Fluid responsiveness is better predicted by dynamic indices of reserve. Changes in pulse pressure or CVP with leg raising suggest more volume will aid, especially in those being mechanically ventilated and in a regular rhythm. Among spontaneously breathing patients, respiratory collapse of the inferior vena cava is another helpful indicator. Minimal IVC variation is associated with supranormal CVP and a low probability of fluid responsiveness. Inspiratory IVC collapse >50% general indicates a patient that is more likely to augment stroke volume with fluid therapy.

Vasopressor Support

Abnormal vasomotor tone and impaired vascular reactivity of sepsis manifest as persistent hypotension despite fluid optimization. *The goal of vasopressor therapy is to restore blood pressure within organ auto-regulatory range.* Fluid optimization is ideally achieved prior to catecholamine support, but patients with severe hemodynamic compromise benefit from early vasopressor support in tandem with ongoing volume resuscitation. *A key error is withholding vasopressor therapy until hemodynamic collapse occurs.* A MAP target of 65 mm Hg is commonly recommended for titrating vasopressors. However, individualized therapy is needed in the face of concomitant or preexisting comorbid disease. As an example, higher perfusion pressure goals may be required to maintain organ blood flow in patients with right shifted auto-regulation due to chronic hypertension. Invasive arterial measurement helps monitoring in patients exhibiting persistent hypotension and requiring catecholamine support.

There is no clear evidence to declare a single superior vasopressor agent. *Norepinephrine is generally considered the first drug of choice* due to its availability, potency, and wide dosing range. Dopamine is also commonly used and has the benefit of cardiac acceleration for patients with inappropriate bradycardia or cardiomyopathy but is associated with more dysrhythmias.[4] There is no role for low-dose "renal" dopamine in attempt to preserve renal function during vasopressor support. Vasodilatory shock is associated with endogenous vasopressin deficiency, which is responsive to vasopressin replacement. Hypotension refractory to typical doses of catecholamine therapy warrants addition of vasopressin. Mortality benefit remains uncertain but vasopressin is safe within the intravenous dosing range of 0.02–0.04 units/minute. Dose escalation is not recommended due to ischemic complications.

Resuscitation Goals

The ultimate goal of resuscitation is to restore oxygen delivery and tissue perfusion to meet metabolic needs. The most appropriate endpoint or target of resuscitation to achieve this goal remains controversial. Historically, resuscitation aimed to normalize clinical markers, but a growing body of evidence shows that resuscitation targeting customary markers of blood pressure, pulse, CVP, and urine output does not guarantee normal organ perfusion. Resuscitation aimed to these targets alone risks leaving the patient in compensated shock.

Central venous oxygen saturation and serum lactate are the best current markers of global perfusion and physiologic stress. Inadequate oxygen delivery is compensated by enhanced tissue extraction and results in desaturation of blood returning to the heart. Mixed (SvO_2) and central venous ($ScvO_2$) oximetry therefore measure the balance between systemic oxygen delivery and consumption. $ScvO_2$ —either continuous via a special catheter or via intermittent blood sampling and measurement of saturation—is *a practical bedside measurement of resuscitation adequacy* that is sampled from a catheter positioned in the superior vena cava. On rare occasions, a normal or elevated $ScvO_2$ can exist despite shock, from either cellular (mitochondrial) dysfunction or shunting. This is why $ScvO_2$ alone cannot be used as "the marker" of resuscitation.

An $ScvO_2$ target of 70% or above was a central management variable in one landmark resuscitation trial and many quasi-experimental follow-up trials.[5] The maximal $ScvO_2$ achieved in the first 6 hours of care is associated with mortality and patients with persistent venous hypoxia experience mortality nearly double that of patients with normalization.[6]

Lactate clearance or trends also aid assessing the response to therapy. A lactate clearance of 10% or more over the first 6 hours of care is associated with improved survival.[7] Targeting lactate clearance (>10%) improves outcomes and was equivalent to targeting $ScvO_2$ as a early resuscitation endpoint.[8]

Unfortunately, *there is no single best endpoint of resuscitation* for all clinical circumstances. Figure 2.1 gives an example of an early sepsis resuscitation protocol. A multimodal approach seeking to normalize a combination of global ($ScvO_2$ and lactate) and regional perfusion markers is likely the best approach. Following urine output and clinical perfusion, parameters remain gauges of resuscitation over hours and should be monitored. Regional perfusion estimation by tissue capnometry, oximetry, and capillary bed microscopy are promising future endpoints of resuscitation, but they are not practical now.

Perfusion Optimization

Cardiac dysfunction is common in patients with severe sepsis as a consequence of chronic disease or acute sepsis-associated cardiomyopathy. Dobutamine is the preferred inotrope to augment cardiac performance. Low-dose initiation (2.5 mcg/kg per minute IV) is recommended to monitor for adverse hypotension

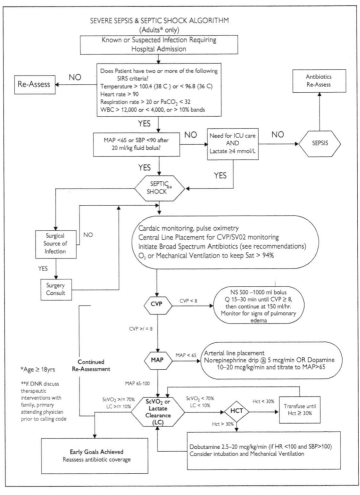

Figure 2.1 Example of an early severe sepsis and septic shock treatment protocol.

or tachycardia with subsequent titration to clinical effect. Milrinone is an alternative choice for patients with tachycardia or prior beta-blocker use.

Augmentation of oxygen carrying capacity via red cell transfusion is an option for patients with persistent oxygen delivery consumption mismatch despite cardiac performance optimization. There is little evidence to declare an optimal hemoglobin threshold for patients with acute severe infection. A restrictive transfusion strategy targeting hemoglobin of 7–9 g/dL is not associated with increased mortality in patients with critical illness. However, patients undergoing acute resuscitation have not been investigated. Red cell transfusion should be considered for critical anemia defined by persistent hypoperfusion despite preload and cardiac performance optimization and hemoglobin <10 g/dL. Serial single unit transfusions are most appropriately guided by the resuscitation targets rather than an arbitrary hemoglobin level. The risk of transfusion-induced lung injury and the limited oxygen delivery abilities of stored blood make aggressive use of uncertain value.

Decreasing systemic oxygen consumption is another potential target of therapy. Respiration and pyrexia are two common sources of enhanced oxygen demand in infected patients—ease either when resuscitation is failing.

Early Infection Control

Source identification and effective infection control are central goals during the early resuscitation of patients with life-threatening infection. Try to collect blood and other culture specimens prior to antibiotics *but do not delay therapy.* Administration of antibiotics within 1 hour of severe sepsis recognition is recommended but often not achieved or feasible.

Empiric coverage should be broad to cover all potential culprit organisms. Inappropriate therapy is associated with five-fold reduction in survival. Patients with resistant (e.g., MRSA, VRE, extended-spectrum beta-lactamase producing gram-negative rods) and atypical organisms are more likely to suffer the consequences of inappropriate empiric therapy. The choice of empiric agents should be individualized per patient drug tolerance, local microbe resistance patterns, suspected source, and host tissue involved.

Anatomic source identification is coupled with consideration of the need for definitive infection control measures. Common foci of infection that are amenable to intervention include peritonitis, intestinal ischemia, cholangitis, pyelonephritis, empyema, indwelling vascular hardware, necrotizing soft-tissue infection, and other deep space infections. Drainage, debridement, and removal of these sources often require coordinated multidisciplinary effort but are part of resuscitation and should not be delayed for the hope of improved cardiovascular stabilization. Percutaneous drainage is generally preferred over open debridement to minimize additional physiologic insult.

Adjunctive Therapies

Inadequate adrenal response in the setting of acute critical illness is termed relative adrenal insufficiency (RAI). Steroid supplementation aims to replace physiologic hormone function in patients suffering from this inadequate reserve. Unfortunately, diagnosis of RAI is limited due to inconsistency of proposed criteria and cortisol immunoassays. Adrenocorticotropic hormone (ACTH) testing is therefore not advised to select infected patients for steroid therapy. *Patients exhibiting fluid and vasopressor-refractory shock are candidates for intravenous steroids.* Hydrocortisone (100–300 mg IV) is the preferred agent, although mortality benefit remains unclear. Stress dose steroids are also indicated for severe sepsis patients with known adrenal dysfunction or chronic steroid dependency even in the absence of shock. Dexamethasone is a suboptimal substitute for hydrocortisone, and high-dose corticosteroids are potentially harmful and not indicated in acute infection.

Polyvalent intravenous immunoglobulin (IVIG) theoretically provides a protective effect in sepsis via several immuno-modulating pathways. To date, pooled analyses fail to provide clear consensus on the role of various IVIG formulations in adult severe sepsis and septic shock. IVIG remains a recommended adjunct in the treatment of streptococcal toxic shock syndrome.

Supportive Therapies

The fragility of critically ill patient mandates detailed attention to routine general care to prevent complications and improve outcomes. Evidence-based support strategies are not specific to the intensive care unit (ICU) and warrant consideration early in care. The current trend of delayed ICU admission due to hospital crowding reinforces the importance of these strategies prior to ICU admission.

Sepsis is the most common cause of acute lung injury (ALI) and these patients often require mechanical ventilatory support. Volume control is the most common mode of ventilation in the absence of evidence pointing to a clearly superior method of support. Adequate gas exchange and lung protection are the overriding principles of ventilator management. In patients with ALI/ARDS, appropriate mechanical ventilation targets both low-tidal volume (TV <7 cc/kg ideal body weight) and plateau airway pressure (<30 cm H_2O).

Prognosis

Accurate prognosis of patient outcome with sepsis remains difficult. Scoring systems that are commonly used in ICUs, such as the acute physiology and chronic health evaluation (APACHE) score, have not gained widespread favor in the ED and require data that are not readily available in the initial hours of care. The mortality in ED sepsis (MEDS) score is an ED-specific scoring system that is useful for predicting outcome from sepsis but has not been shown to be useful in prognosis of patients with septic shock.[9]

The most reliable and useful measure of prognosis is the number and severity of failed organs. Thus, the sequential organ failure assessment (SOFA) score is a readily available and easy-to-use indicator of sepsis severity in the ED.[10] The initial SOFA score is of less value than the trend, which provides information on progression or resolution of organ dysfunction.

Pearls of Care

1. Sepsis is common in the ED and is associated with high morbidity and mortality.
2. Lactate is a useful biomarker to confirm and risk-stratify critical illness, including in sepsis.
3. Early recognition of severe sepsis is critical and must be coupled to timely and effective therapy to improve outcome.
4. A multimodal, quantitative approach to resuscitation that seeks to normalize a combination of global (ScvO$_2$ and lactate) and regional perfusion markers is likely the best approach.
5. Norepinephrine is the vasopressor of choice due to its availability, potency, and wide dosing range.

References

1. Marchick MR, Kline JA, Jones AE. The significance of non-sustained hypotension in emergency department patients with sepsis. *Intensive Care Med* 2009;35:1261–1264.
2. Howell MD, Donnino M, Clardy P, Talmor D, Shapiro NI. Occult hypoperfusion and mortality in patients with suspected infection. *Intensive Care Med* 2007;33:1892–1899.
3. Jones AE, Brown MD, Trzeciak S, et al. The effect of a quantitative resuscitation strategy on mortality in patients with sepsis: a meta-analysis. *Crit Care Med* 2008;36:2734–2739.
4. De Backer D., Biston P, Devriendt J, et al. Comparison of dopamine and norepinephrine in the treatment of shock. *New Engl J Med* 2010;362:779–789.
5. Rivers E, Nguyen B, Havstad S, et al. Early goal-directed therapy in the treatment of severe sepsis and septic shock. *N Engl J Med* 2001;345:1368–1377.
6. Pope JV, Jones AE, Gaieski DF, Arnold RC, Trzeciak S, Shapiro NI. Multicenter study of central venous oxygen saturation (ScvO(2)) as a predictor of mortality in patients with sepsis. *Ann Emerg Med* 2010;55:40–46.
7. Arnold RC, Shapiro NI, Jones AE, et al. Multi-center study of early lactate clearance as a determinant of survival in patients with presumed sepsis. *Shock* 2009;32:36–39.
8. Jones AE, Shapiro NI, Trzeciak S, et al. Lactate clearance vs central venous oxygen saturation as goals of early sepsis therapy: a randomized clinical trial. *JAMA* 2010;303:739–746.
9. Shapiro N, Wolfe R, Moore R, Smith E, Burdick E, Bates D. Mortality in Emergency Department Sepsis (MEDS) score: a prospectively derived and validated clinical prediction rule. *Crit Care Med* 2003;31:670–675.
10. Jones AE, Trzeciak S, Kline JA. The Sequential Organ Failure Assessment score for predicting outcome in patients with severe sepsis and evidence of hypoperfusion at the time of emergency department presentation. *Crit Care Med* 2009;37:1649–1654.

Chapter 3

Respiratory Failure (Including Parenchymal, Vascular, and Central Causes)

David F. Gaieski and Munish Goyal

Introduction

The incidence of respiratory failure in patients presenting to the emergency department (ED) has not been well characterized and will vary significantly depending upon the disease severity of the patient population for any given ED. Similarly, the mortality from respiratory failure varies depending upon the cause and can be as high as 45% in patients with acute respiratory distress syndrome (ARDS). Recognition and initial management of respiratory failure are fundamental tasks of the emergency physician (EP). While simple in theory, optimal diagnosis and intervention can be difficult and complex in the ED. Respiratory failure occurs when the patient fails to perform one or both of the primary gas exchange processes: oxygenation and ventilation. Respiratory failure results from parenchymal, vascular, or central causes. Respiratory failure may be acute, chronic, or acute on chronic. Appropriate interventions differ substantially depending upon the primary etiology. Respiratory failure may be defined as present when a patient cannot maintain an arterial PaO_2 >60 mm Hg or an arterial $PaCO_2$ <50 mm Hg.

Patients with evolving or impending respiratory failure often present to the ED in acute distress, which limits the history obtainable from and physical examination of these patients. Clinical decisions may need to be made based on a limited data set and without blood gas values. Initial data should include a rapid visual evaluation of the patient: what are the patient's mental status, body position, and respiratory effort? What are the patient's vital signs, including temperature, blood pressure, heart rate, and respiratory rate? Pulse oximetry should be immediately obtained, and the heart and lungs should be auscultated. From this information, the EP must decide whether the patient is in acute respiratory failure, in respiratory distress with impending failure, has a significant potential for progression to respiratory failure, or appears to be stable without initial signs of respiratory failure. Immediate management will depend upon the findings from this brief, initial evaluation. When a patient presents with significantly decreased mental status, not protecting his or her airway, and with minimal or no respiratory effort, securing the patient's airway to decrease the risk of aspiration and ensure adequate breathing takes precedence over other basic tasks. In other clinical scenarios, the clinician has time to perform additional tasks before definitive airway management occurs.

Definition of Terms

Acute lung injury (ALI): lung damage not associated with cardiogenic pulmonary edema resulting in bilateral infiltrates on chest radiograph and a PaO_2/FiO_2 (P/F) ratio <300.

Acute respiratory distress syndrome (ARDS): lung damage not associated with cardiogenic pulmonary edema resulting in bilateral infiltrates on chest radiograph and a P/F ratio <200.

Diffusion: the ability of oxygen to cross over the alveolar membrane from the alveolar space to the pulmonary vasculature and be bound by hemoglobin, along with the ability of carbon dioxide to diffuse from the blood to the alveoli to be eliminated from the body.

Hypercapnia: $PaCO_2$ >50 mm Hg on room air.

Hypoxemia: PaO_2 <60 mm Hg on room air (see Table 3.1).

Inadequate perfusion: regional or generalized inadequate blood flow through the pulmonary vasculature to maintain gas exchange.

Inadequate ventilation: insufficient respiratory performance to promote gas exchange, usually leading to hypercapnia, sometimes associated with hypoxemia.

P/F ratio: the ratio of the partial pressure of arterial oxygen (PaO_2) to the fractional proportion of oxygen in the inspired gas (FiO_2). This ratio is used to assess lung oxygenation performance.

Respiratory failure: inadequate gas exchange in the lungs such that arterial oxygen level falls (hypoxemia) and/or arterial carbon dioxide level rises (hypercapnia) and these values can no longer be maintained in the normal range.

Clinical Syndromes (Both Symptom and Organ Based)

Respiratory failure can be divided into acute and chronic respiratory failure. A central task for the clinician is to differentiate between the two and

Table 3.1 Five Primary Causes of Hypoxemia
1 Low fraction of oxygen in inspired air
2 Alveolar hypoventilation
3 Defects in diffusion
4 Ventilation/perfusion mismatch
5 Shunt

to understand when an acute component is superimposed upon a chronic baseline. Acute respiratory failure can be further divided into hypoxemic and hypercapnic (also known as Type I and Type II, respectively), depending upon the basic presentation and underlying pathology. Hypoxemic respiratory failure is characterized by a PaO_2 <60 mm Hg and, usually, by a low or normal $PaCO_2$. Hypoxemic respiratory failure can be caused by parenchymal, vascular, or central abnormalities. Hypercapnic respiratory failure is characterized by a $PaCO_2$ >50 mm Hg and, usually, by a low PaO_2 if the patient is breathing room air. Hypercapnic respiratory failure can be caused by severe problems with airflow (asthma, chronic obstructive pulmonary disease [COPD]), hypoventilation (obesity hypoventilation syndrome, chest wall injuries), and central causes, including drug overdoses.

Symptom Based

Dyspnea: Dyspnea, which can be defined as difficulty breathing or shortness of breath, is the cardinal symptom of respiratory failure in patients who can communicate their perception of their disease.

Chest pain: Chest pain is a common accompanying symptom in patients with impending or full-blown respiratory failure. Chest pain can be from pleural irritation, chest wall trauma, myocardial ischemia, or a more generalized discomfort associated with air hunger.

Sign Based

Fever: When respiratory failure occurs in the setting of severe sepsis, patients often present with a fever. Respiratory failure is often associated with tachypnea and mouth breathing, which may lower the measured oral temperature. The clinician should strongly consider obtaining a core temperature (rectal, esophageal, bladder) in the undifferentiated patient with respiratory failure.

Tachypnea: An increased respiratory rate is one of the hallmarks of hypoxemic respiratory failure.

Bradypnea: Patients with hypercapnic respiratory failure, especially when caused by central pathology or overdoses, can present with a markedly decreased respiratory rate.

Tachycardia: Hypoxemia is a potent trigger of catecholamine release, and tachycardia is often present in patients with respiratory failure.

Hypertension: Since hypoxemia is a potent trigger of catecholamine release, hypertension is also often present in patients with respiratory failure.

Altered mental status: Hypoxemia and hypercapnia may alter global level of consciousness. Hypoxemia is associated with agitation or somnolence. Hypercapnia is associated with somnolence, myoclonic jerking, seizures, and coma. In addition, many central causes of respiratory failure, including intracranial hemorrhage (ICH), cerebrovascular accidents (CVA), and drug overdoses, are accompanied by decreased mental status.

Cyanosis: Hypoxemia is associated with cyanosis, particularly of the lips and nailbeds.

Organ Based

Parenchymal: Parenchymal causes of respiratory failure include problems in the transmitting airways, alveoli, and lung parenchyma. These include asthma, COPD, pneumothorax, obstruction, pneumonia, and ALI/ARDS. These conditions are characterized by the presence of ventilation/perfusion (V/Q) mismatch where there is an imbalance between ventilation and perfusion, and areas of low ventilation relative to perfusion produce low levels of oxygen diffusion, resulting in hypoxemia.

Vascular: Vascular causes of respiratory failure include pump dysfunction, pulmonary embolism, cardiac tamponade, and vascular shunts. Examples of pump dysfunction include congestive heart failure or cardiogenic shock, resulting in inadequate blood flow to maintain gas exchange. Pulmonary embolism leads to decreased blood flow through the pulmonary vasculature and creates significant V/Q mismatch,

Central: Central causes of respiratory failure include drug overdoses resulting in central depression of respiratory drive (e.g., opioid overdoses), central nervous system trauma, ICH, CVA, and a variety of causes of encephalopathy (septic, hepatic, or hypertensive).

General and Key Management Principles and Controversies

Establish a Definitive Airway Quickly when there is Uncertainty about Patency of Airway or Adequacy of Ventilation

When a patient presents with full-blown or impending respiratory failure, the EP must make rapid, critical decisions, often with limited information. If at any point in the evaluation and treatment the patient is *in extremis*, is not protecting his or her airway, or has agonal respirations, immediate placement of an endotracheal tube and establishment of mechanical ventilation should occur. Exceptions to this include when the respiratory arrest is of sudden onset or related to cardiac arrest of obvious cardiac etiology. In this case, definitive airway management is delayed for several minutes during initial cardiopulmonary resuscitation, prioritizing defibrillation, chest compressions, and drug delivery over definitive airway management.

Supplemental Therapies during Initiation of Mechanical Ventilation

Many patients are extremely unstable at the time they are placed on mechanical ventilation. If attention is not paid to details of patient management during the transition from spontaneous to mechanical ventilation, the patient can decompensate further. Preoxygenation with 100% FiO_2 should be used whenever possible to replace residual nitrogen with oxygen. In patients with profound hypoxemia who are protecting their airway, the clinician may consider using noninvasive positive pressure ventilation (NIPPV) to improve oxygen reserve as a bridge to intubation. This allows for more time to establish a definitive airway without continued hypoxemia. In addition, some patients may require a bolus of fluid prior to intubation to support their blood pressure, because the catecholamine surge triggered by hypoxemia will be blunted by the induction and paralytic agents used during rapid sequence intubation (RSI). Patients with hypoxemic respiratory failure often present to the ED multiple days into their disease process and are volume depleted secondary to extensive insensible fluid losses from tachypnea and decreased oral fluid intake. In addition to aggressive fluid resuscitation, some patients may require a bolus dose of vasopressor (consider phenylephrine 50 mcg) during RSI. In other patients, especially those with severe sepsis, where respiratory failure occurs in the setting of metabolic acidosis, a period of NIPPV can help increase the patient's minute ventilation, improve oxygenation prior to endotracheal intubation, and guide initial ventilator settings to maintain adequate acid-base status.

Reevaluate Etiology Based on Response to Treatment

Different causes of respiratory failure can be difficult to distinguish at the most proximal point of presentation even though initial treatment approaches may be diametrically opposed. For example, a middle-aged patient with a history of congestive heart failure may present with several days of progressive dyspnea and chest pain. The history is limited by the patient's critical illness. On initial evaluation, she is found to be hypertensive, tachycardic, tachypneic, and markedly hypoxemic. Lung exam reveals diffuse crackles. Emergent chest radiography reveals diffuse pulmonary edema. At this point, the clinician needs to decide on initial therapeutic interventions. If the clinician decides to implement high-flow oxygen, noninvasive positive pressure ventilation (NIPPV), and vasodilator and diuretic therapy, monitoring of the clinical response to these interventions is essential. For example, if the cause of the patient's presentation was acute decompensated heart failure, the patient may experience improved oxygenation, decreased work of breathing, and become more comfortable with normalization of vital signs after the aforementioned interventions. Conversely, if the clinical presentation was the result of severe influenza pneumonia and resultant ARDS, the patient may respond to the aforementioned interventions by becoming hypotensive, more tachypneic and tachycardic, and have minimal improvement in oxygenation. Only through continual reassessment of the patient and reconsideration of the etiology of respiratory failure will the clinician be able to understand these responses to therapy and modify the management strategy to best treat the patient.

Management of Respiratory Failure Does Not Stop with the Establishment of a Definitive Airway

Successful placement of a definitive airway is only the beginning of an EP's management of a patient with respiratory failure. After the endotracheal tube is secured and placement is confirmed (capnography, auscultation, chest radiography), further interventions to address the cause of respiratory failure are

Table 3.2 Interventions to Improve Gas Exchange

Interventions to Decrease PaCO$_2$ (Increase minute ventilation)
Increase respiratory rate
Increase tidal volume
Prolong inspiratory time (inspiratory: expiratory ratio)
Interventions to Increase PaO$_2$
Increase FiO$_2$
Increase PEEP
Increase mean airway pressure (bilevel or other regimens)
Correct parenchymal dysfunction (pulmonary edema)
Correct ventilation-perfusion mismatch (recruit collapsed lung, remove mucous plugs, etc.)
Interventions to Decrease High Peak Pressures
Decrease tidal volume
Prolong expiratory time
Increase sedation and paralyze patient
Pressure-controlled ventilation

mandatory. For example, patients with respiratory failure related to massive pulmonary embolism are usually preload dependent, requiring volume infusion to maintain adequate cardiac filling, and need to be treated with anticoagulants or with thrombolytic agents.

Ventilator Management is a Key Task of Emergency Physicians

An endotracheal tube is not a therapy in and of itself; rather, it establishes a secure connection between the patient and a mechanical ventilator, which will deliver the primary therapy to improve the patient's respiratory failure. Ventilator settings need to be chosen depending upon the cause of respiratory failure. EPs are obliged to develop sophisticated strategies geared toward initial ventilator management (Table 3.2). For example, a young, healthy patient who is intubated for airway protection in the setting of acute alcohol toxicity requires very different ventilator settings from a septic shock patient who is intubated to decrease the work of breathing associated with profound lactic acidosis. There are two basic goals of ED ventilator management. The first is manipulating ventilator settings to maintain a PaO$_2$ >60 mm Hg, with rapid titration of FiO$_2$ to the minimal required level to avoid extended periods of arterial and alveolar hyperoxia. The second consists of manipulations to decrease PaCO$_2$ to <50 mm Hg or a level where the arterial pH is normalized, if conditions permit.

Noninvasive Positive Pressure Ventilation Can Be the Initial Strategy in a Significant Percentage of Patients with Respiratory Failure from a Reversible Cause

In patients where acute respiratory failure occurs from a rapidly reversible cause and their respiratory drive is maintained, a trial of NIPPV may be appropriate. Many patients who present to the ED in undifferentiated respiratory failure with an active respiratory drive and are able to follow commands are candidates for NIPPV. Contraindications include airway obstruction, active vomiting, or grossly uncooperative patients.

Data support the use of NIPPV for patients suffering from acute exacerbations of chronic obstructive pulmonary disease (COPD). A Cochrane review published in 2003 associated NIPPV with lower mortality, lower need for intubation, lower likelihood of treatment failure, shorter duration of hospitalization, and greater improvements at 1 hour in pH, $PaCO_2$, and respiratory rate when compared to usual medical care. The authors suggest that NIPPV should be part of the first-line intervention to manage respiratory failure secondary to an acute exacerbation of COPD and that application of NIPPV should occur early.

Acute cardiogenic pulmonary edema (ACPE) is a less well-accepted indication for NIPPV. A recent, large meta-analysis compared treatment approaches for patients with ACPE. When compared to standard oxygen therapy, NIPPV reduced mortality and need for intubation. Because of its potential efficacy, a trial of NIPPV can be utilized in patients with hypercapnic respiratory failure secondary to COPD or ACPE who present with depressed mental status, as long as they have preserved work of breathing. These patients require close observation and frequent reassessment to gauge efficacy of therapy.

Noninvasive positive pressure ventilation has also been shown to be effective in patients who suffer acute asthma exacerbations or are immunocompromised and develop pneumonia. During the workup, if it's determined that the patient will require endotracheal intubation, then initiation of NIPPV prior to RSI will reduce arterial hypoxemia during and after intubation as compared to preoxygenation with a nonrebreather bag-valve mask.

Emergency Department Ventilator Strategies Impact on Outcomes in Critically Ill Patients Intubated in the Emergency Department

There are emerging data to suggest that ED management of patients intubated for acute respiratory failure impacts long-term outcomes, including development of ventilator-associated pneumonia (VAP), ALI, ARDS, organ failure, and mortality. For example, ED length of stay is an independent risk factor for development of VAP in emergently intubated blunt trauma patients (see Fig. 3.1). Accepted VAP prevention interventions are rarely performed in the ED, but it is recommended that intensive care unit (ICU) standard-of-care procedures be implemented as soon as possible. These include elevation of the head of the bed, oral care and suctioning of subglottic secretions. There is also a strong association between the initial tidal volume selected for mechanical ventilation and the subsequent development of ALI. Risk of ALI increases for each 1 mL/kg tidal volume greater than the 6 mL/kg used in the lung preservation arm of the ARDSNet trial. Therefore, it may be important to limit large tidal volumes for patients with ALI and also in patients at risk for ALI.

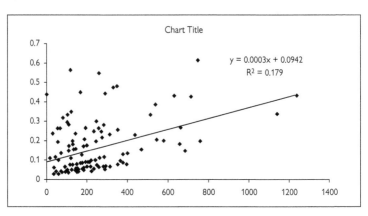

Figure 3.1 Emergency department length of stay (minutes) (x axis) versus probability of ventilator-associated pneumonia (y axis).

Pearls of Care

1. Respiratory failure is present when a patient cannot achieve an arterial PaO_2 >60 mm Hg or maintain a $PaCO_2$ <50 mm Hg.
2. Anticipate and correct peri-intubation hypotension with fluid boluses and infusions or boluses of vasopressors.
3. Endotracheal intubation is part of the definitive initial management of respiratory failure by providing an interface between the patient and a mechanical ventilator.
4. Noninvasive positive pressure ventilation should be considered early in undifferentiated respiratory failure if the patient has a respiratory drive and is following commands. Noninvasive positive pressure ventilation can serve as a bridge to endotracheal intubation.
5. Early implementation of ICU ventilator strategies can contribute to improved outcomes and prevent complications, including ARDS and VAP.

Selected Readings

Acute Respiratory Distress Syndrome Network. Ventilation with lower tidal volumes as compared with traditional tidal volumes for acute lung injury and the acute respiratory distress syndrome. The Acute Respiratory Distress Syndrome Network. *N Engl J Med* 2000;342(18):1301–1308.

Andrews P, Azoulay E, Antonelli M, et al. Year in review in intensive care medicine. 2005. I. Acute respiratory failure and acute lung injury, ventilation, hemodynamics, education, renal failure. *Intensive Care Med* 2006;32(2):207–216

Carr BG, Kaye A, Wiebe DJ, et al. Emergency department length of stay: a major risk factor for pneumonia in intubated blunt trauma patients. *J Trauma*. 2007;63:9–12.

Chonghaile MN, Higgins B, Laffey JG. Permissive hypercapnia: role in lung protective strategies. *Curr Opinion Crit Care* 2005;11:56–62.

Gajic O, Frutos-Vivar E, Esteban A, et al. Ventilator settings as a risk factor for acute respiratory distress syndrome in mechanically ventilated patients. *Int Care Med* 2005;31:922–926.

Girard TD, Kress JP, Fuchs BD, et al. Efficacy and safety of a paired sedation and ventilator weaning protocol for mechanically ventilated patients in intensive care (awake and breathing controlled trial): a randomized controlled trial *Lancet*. 2008;371:126–134.

Gray A, Goodacre S, Newby DE, et al. Non-invasive ventilation in acute cardiogenic pulmonary edema. *New Engl J Med*. 2008;359:142–151.

Lightowler JV, Wedzicha JA, Elliott MW, et al. Noninvasive positive pressure ventilation to treat respiratory failure resulting from exacerbations of chronic obstructive pulmonary disease: Cochrane systematic review and metaanalysis. *BMJ* 2003;326:1–5.

Phua J, Badia JR, Adhikari NK, et al. Has mortality from acute respiratory distress syndrome decreased over time? A systematic review. *Am J Respir Crit Care Med* 2009;179(3):220–227.

Weng C-L, Zhao Y-T, Liu Q-H, et al. Meta-analysis: noninvasive ventilation in acute cardiogenic pulmonary edema. *Ann Int Med* 2010;152:590–600.

Chapter 4

Acute Heart Failure

Tertius Tuy and William Frank Peacock

Introduction

Heart failure (HF) is increasingly common. The current prevalence in America is 5 million cases, and its yearly incidence is more than 500,000. It is a disease that favors the elderly, who generally have multiple HF risk factors. Of those hospitalized with HF, about 80% are over the age of 65. Furthermore, HF accounts for 2%–3% of all hospital admissions and approximately 80% of HF patients present at the emergency department (ED).

Overall, patients with HF have a poor prognosis. The 30-day readmission rates for HF increase with advancing age and can be as high as 20%–30%. For acute HF patients, the in-hospital mortality rate ranges widely, with figures as low as 4% and increasing to 60% if shock is present. After the first hospitalization, the 1-year mortality of those with HF is 20%, increasing to over 50% at 5 years.[1]

Definition of Terms

Acute decompensated heart failure (ADHF): a new or worsened HF with signs and symptoms that require medical therapy and/or hospitalization (Table 4.1).

Cardiogenic shock (CS): an extreme form of ADHF where cardiac output is so low that end-organ function is profoundly impaired despite adequate intravascular volume.

Heart failure (HF): this exists when cardiac function cannot provide the needed output to support demand.

Clinical Syndrome

Etiology

Several causes of HF exist (Table 4.2). Decompensation occurs when patients with a background of impaired myocardial function are challenged by various stressors (acute myocardial infarction, uncontrolled hypertension, arrhythmia,

Table 4.1 Clinical Conditions of Acute Heart Failure Syndrome

ADHF (de novo or decompensated chronic heart failure)	• Signs and symptoms of AHF • Do not fulfill criteria of cardiogenic shock, acute pulmonary edema, hypertensive crisis
Hypertensive AHF	• Signs and symptoms of AHF • High BP • Relatively preserved LV function • CXR compatible with acute pulmonary edema
Pulmonary edema	• CXR compatible with acute pulmonary edema • Severe respiratory distress • Crackles over the lungs • Orthopnea • O_2 < 90% on room air
Cardiogenic shock	• Evidence of tissue hypoperfusion • Reduced BP (SBP <90 mm Hg or drop of arterial BP by >30 mm Hg) • Low urine output (< 0.5 mL/kg per hour) • Pulse rate >60 bpm
High output failure	• Tachycardia • Warm peripheries • Pulmonary congestion • ± Low BP
RHF	• Low CO • Increase JVD • Hepatomegaly • Hypotension

ADHF, acute decompensated heart failure; AHF, acute heart failure; BP, blood pressure; CO, cardiac output; JVD, jugular venous distension; RHF, renal heart failure; SBP, systolic blood pressure.

etc.). The most common etiology of CS is acute myocardial infarction (AMI) with left ventricular failure, followed by acute mitral regurgitation, acute ventricular septal defect, isolated right ventricle infarct, and tamponade.[2]

Pathophysiology

Cardiac dysfunction results in diminished cardiac output (CO) and elevated filling pressures. The increased filling pressures are reflected by elevated central venous pressures (CVP). Pulmonary edema occurs when the left ventricular filling pressures propagate into the pulmonary vasculature and creates hypoxemia, acidosis, and further dysfunction.

As CVP increases and CO decreases, renal perfusion declines. The drop in renal perfusion is a result of activation of the neurohormonal system (NHS) and its downstream mediators, which include the renin-angiotensin-aldosterone-system (RAAS), the sympathetic nervous system (SNS), and the endothelin system (ET-1).

Table 4.2 Major Etiologies of Heart Failure
1. Coronary artery disease
2. Complications of myocardial infarction
• Acute mitral regurgitation (papillary rupture)
• Cardiac free wall rupture
3. Sustained cardiac arrhythmia/tachycardia
4. Poorly controlled hypertension
5. Valvular rupture or disease
6. Myocarditis
7. Idiopathic cardiomyopathy
8. Postpartum cardiomyopathy
9. Acute pulmonary embolus
10. Pericardial disease/tamponade
• Effusion
• Constrictive pericarditis
11. Hyperkinetic states
• Anemia
• Thyrotoxicosis
• A-V fistula (e.g., dialysis)

With a 25% impairment of systolic contraction, acute heart failure may occur; at 40%, cardiogenic shock is imminent. With preexisting heart failure, even minor cardiac ischemia can trigger CS.

Systolic Heart Failure versus Diastolic Heart Failure

Systolic heart failure results from diminished myocardial contractility, usually with an ejection fraction less than 40%. When stressed, the cardiac function is incapable of responding and intracardiac pressures rise, resulting in dyspnea, fatigue, or pulmonary edema.

Diastolic heart failure (also called "HF with preserved systolic function") is the inability of the heart to relax. Cardiac compliance is decreased while end-diastolic pressures are increased and systemic hypertension may be present. Transmission of these pressures to the pulmonary and systemic vasculature results in the congestive symptoms similarly seen with systolic dysfunction. The ejection fraction is preserved in diastolic HF at or above 40%.

History

Patients with ADHF commonly present with shortness of breath. Table 4.3 provides a list of other common symptoms and complaints.[3,10] Previous heart failure, ventricular dysfunction, or myocardial infarction are strong predictors that the new dyspnea or weakness is likely from ADHF.

Severe ADHF patients may complain of fatigue, nausea, symptoms of hypotension, altered mental status, or less urine output. In CS there are profound

Table 4.3 Common Symptoms of Acute Decompensated Heart Failure

Symptoms	Presentation (%)
Dyspnea	87–93
Exertional	86–97
Orthopnea	10–59
Paroxysmal nocturnal dyspnea	13–39
At rest	1–6
Fatigue	17–56
Weight gain	5–15
Cough	3–51
Chest discomfort	28–37
Edema	35–70
Nausea/vomiting	8–17

or multiple signs of reduced cardiac output (hypotension), tissue hypoperfusion (little urine output or cool skin), or volume overload (dyspnea at rest, rales).

Physical Exam

Assess the airway first for patency, then evaluate the circulation, with hypotension or a pulse pressure <20 mm Hg being indicative of potential CS.

Tachypnea is common until late stages where respiratory fatigue occurs. Hypoperfusion may cause the extremities to be pale, cool, or mottled. The neck may show jugular venous distention (JVD) from decreased right ventricular and venous compliance. Vascular congestion may cause gravity-dependent pitting edema and hepatomegaly.

Auscultation of the lungs may reveal rales from interstitial edema or diminished breath sounds secondary to pleural effusions. In right ventricular infarct, the lung fields may be clear despite having JVD since LV function remains intact.

Presence of an S3 gallop has a PPV of 95% and a NPV of 32% for an EF <50%. Suspect mechanical dysfunction if there is a new onset of a systolic murmur. Papillary muscle dysfunction or chordae tendinea rupture will produce an acute mitral regurgitation (MR). A new loud holosystolic ejection murmur heard loudest at the left parasternal edge of the precordium may indicate a new ventricular septal defect (VSD).

Since ADHF is a syndrome without a single gold standard diagnostic test, it can be difficult to diagnose at the initial presentation. The Framingham criteria (Table 4.4), using history and physical findings, require at least one major and two minor criteria for diagnosis. The Boston criteria (Table 4.4), adds chest X-ray (CXR) to the history and exam. More points give higher probabilities for HF. A score ≥ 4 correlates with a pulmonary artery occlusion pressure ≥ 12 mm Hg and has a sensitivity and specificity of 90% and 85%, respectively. While individual physical findings are often unreliable, *the overall gestalt by an experienced clinician is accurate 85% of the time.*

Differential Diagnosis

Many other conditions can mimic ADHF, including pulmonary embolus (PE), chronic obstructive pulmonary disease (COPD) exacerbation, pneumonia, and acute pulmonary edema.

Diagnostic Tools

Electrocardiogram

While not diagnostic for ADHF, the electrocardiogram may identify ischemia or infarction by ST segment, or Q- or T-wave changes. *Any new ischemia on electrocardiogram (ECG) correlates to higher short-term ADHF mortality and morbidity.* Chronic heart failure and hypertension may show cardiac strain, atrial hypertrophy, ventricular hypertrophy, or dilated cardiomyopathy.

Chest Radiography

The sensitivity of the CXR is dependent on timing, position of the patient, the view, severity of HF, and concurrent comorbidities. The absence of radiographic signs does not exclude abnormal LV function.[25] Clinical findings may precede any radiographic findings by hours, but *patients with profound breathing symptoms rarely have normal radiographs.* In mild HF, dilated upper lobe vessels alone are found in >60% of patients. The presence of cardiomegaly, a sign of chronic remodeling, has poor sensitivity.

Laboratory

The natriuretic peptides (NPs), B-type natriuretic peptide (BNP) or its inactive precursor NT-proBNP, can assist in differentiating patients with suspected HF from other causes of dyspnea.[4] They are best used when uncertain and not routinely, and other primary events can raise these levels (notably acute pulmonary embolism, pneumonia, or acute obstructive lung disease—each causes some RV strain).

When NPs are markedly elevated (>500 pg/mL BNP or >900 pg/mL NTproBNP), their positive predictive value for diagnosing HF is 90% or above; however, these are rarely "unexpected" findings. When low (<100 pg/mL BNP or <300 pg/mL NTproBNP), consider an alternative diagnosis to primary ADHF. The "gray zone" (100 to 500 pg/mL for BNP, 300 to 900 pg/mL for NTproBNP) NP values demand additional testing and clinical integration to accurately determine ADHF presence or absence. For example, any myocardial stress (e.g., AMI, pulmonary embolus) may elevate natriuretic peptides, along with renal failure and cirrhosis. Alternatively, obesity may lower BNP levels, resulting in an inverse relationship between the NP level and body mass index.

While increased natriuretic peptide levels correlate with increased short-term mortality, it is unclear what new prognostic information these add. The Acute Decompensated Heart Failure Registry (ADHERE) noted that patients with a BNP >1730 pg/mL at ED presentation had a 6% in-hospital mortality compared

Table 4.4 Criteria for the Diagnosis of Heart Failure

Framingham Criteria

Major Criteria
Paroxysmal nocturnal dyspnea
Neck vein distention or hepatojugular reflux
Rales or acute pulmonary edema
Cardiomegaly or S_3 gallop

Minor Criteria
Extremity edema
Dyspnea on exertion or night cough
Hepatomegaly or pleural effusion
Vital capacity reduce by one-third
Tachycardia (≥ 120)

Boston Criteria

History		Physical		Chest X-ray	
Dyspnea at rest	4	S3 gallop	3	Alveolar pulmonary edema	4
Orthopnea or hepatomegaly	4	JVD plus edema	3	Interstitial pulmonary edema	3
Paroxysmal nocturnal dyspnea (PND)	3	Wheezing	3	Bilateral pleural effusions	3
Dyspnea while walking	2	Rales > basilar	2	Cardiothoracic ratio >0.5	3
Dyspnea while climbing stairs	1	JVD >6 cm H_2O	2	Kerley A lines	2
		HR >110 bpm 2			
		HR 91–119 bpm 1			
		Basilar rales 1			

HR, heart rate; JVD, jugular venous distension; PND, paroxysmal nocturnal dyspnea.

to those with a BNP level <430 pg/mL, whose in-hospital mortality rate was 2.2%.[5] How this adds to bedside assessment of risk is uncertain.

Cardiac necrosis markers may aid in determining diagnosis and prognosis of ADHF. Elevated troponin levels (like new ECG ischemic changes) indicate myocardial damage or severe stress and correlate to higher in-hospital mortality.[5, 6]

Other lab investigations may be helpful for prognosis (complete blood count, electrolytes, and renal function) but are not central to ADHF diagnosis. Arterial blood gas may show carbon dioxide retention, hypoxemia, and acidosis. In first-time ADHF, thyroid-stimulating hormone levels may detect thyroid triggers of HF. Serum lactate levels may be helpful in detecting subtle forms of hypoperfusion and CS.

Echocardiogram

Echocardiography allows for the visualization of chamber size, contractility, pericardial fluid, and valve status. While helpful, echocardiography is often difficult to obtain in the ED setting, especially with severe ADHF. It is best used when competing diagnoses are present and to assess ventricular function.

Management of the ABCs

For moderately distressed patients, start oxygen therapy via nasal canula, ventimask, or non-rebreather mask. For patients with severe distress or respiratory fatigue, noninvasive ventilation by biphasic positive airway pressures or continuous positive airway pressure is an option.[7] Endotracheal intubation is reserved for those with severe symptoms, altered sensorium, or who fail the previous therapies. When using any form of positive-pressure ventilation, anticipate a potential drop in blood pressure (BP) from altered venous return. This may require a fluid bolus in the absence of pulmonary congestion or vasopressor therapy.

Once the airway and breathing are secured, the systolic BP (SBP) is best kept at the low end of normal as long as neurological function and urine output are maintained. If the patient is unstable or CS is suspected, cardiac monitoring, central venous access, and an arterial line may make care easier to deliver. Urinary catheterization will allow for assessment of urine production and help track response to therapy, but it is reserved for the most symptomatic patients. More invasive hemodynamic monitoring (e.g., pulmonary artery catheterization) is rarely deployed in the ED.

Management of "Vascular Failure"

Half of the patients with ADHF will present with an elevated SBP (>140 mm Hg), occasionally referred to as "vascular failure." These patients typically have an acute onset of breathlessness. Pulmonary congestion is a result of improper fluid distribution rather than retention of fluids. Therefore, *rapid vasodilator treatment is first-line therapy.*

Currently used vasodilators are nitroglycerin and nitroprusside. Sublingual nitroglycerin may be used first and continued until intravenous access is established. Clinical and hemodynamic response to therapy may be obvious within minutes. Subsequent vasodilator therapy may be added via topical (mild symptoms) or intravenous infusions (more severe symptoms). Even with doses as large as 20,000 mcg of nitroglycerin over 30 minutes, hypotension occurs in <5%. If hypotension occurs, stop the infusion and consider right ventricular myocardial infarction, PE, or sepsis as possible etiologies.

At infusion rates of 30 to 40 mcg/min, nitroglycerin has predominantly venodilatory effects; at higher doses, notably above 250 mcg/min, there is an added arterial dilation. Starting doses of IV nitroglycerin are 10–50 mcg/min, titrated by increments of 10–20 mcg based on symptoms, BP, and PCWP (if used). Tachyphylaxis can occur within 1 to 2 hours of administration, especially with higher doses.

Nitroprusside causes both arterial and venous dilation. Intravenous dosing starts at 10 mcg/min and is titrated upward by 10 mcg/min. Complications are hypotension and cyanide toxicity, the latter is uncommon in the absence of liver or kidney failure.

Nesiritide is recombinant B-type natriuretic peptide that causes venodilation and arterial dilation. It also increases stroke volume and cardiac output, decreases PCWP, and improves both natriuresis and diuresis. It is *not* currently recommended for use because of safety concerns.

Management of "Cardiac Failure"

In the remaining ADHF patients, the SBP is between 90 mm Hg and 140 mm Hg, sometimes referred to as "cardiac failure." The general presentation is a gradual and progressive congestion and breathlessness. *Diuresis is the first-line therapy*, with loop diuretics being the most commonly used agent of volume reduction. Complications include hypotension, electrolyte abnormalities, renal dysfunction, and maladaptive neurohormonal activation. The lowest effective dose of diuretics should be given to minimize adverse events. Furosemide is the most common loop diuretic started, using an intravenous (IV) dose equal to the outpatient oral dose or (in naïve patients) 40 mg IV.

Although β-blockers, angiotensin converting enzyme (ACE) inhibitors, angiotensin II receptor blockers (ARB), and aldosterone antagonists reduce mortality in chronic heart failure, their benefit in initial ADHF care is uncertain. They are contraindicated if there is hypotension, bradycardia, hyperkalemia, or cardiogenic shock.

Historically, morphine sulfate was used to reduce dyspnea and calm the patient. It causes venodilation and mildly decreases preload. In one large registry, morphine use was associated with increased in-hospital mortality; however, the design could not determine a causal relationship, and it is likely that those receiving morphine differed from those not receiving it. The best approach now is to use this judiciously and not as a primary agent to treat ADHF, deploying small boluses (2–5 mg IV) if needed.

Management of Cardiogenic Shock

For ADHF patients and SBP <100 mmHg, CS is likely, and more aggressive treatment is warranted. In the absence of any signs of pulmonary congestion, give a 250 mL normal saline fluid challenge. If pulmonary congestion exists, withhold fluid and give an inotrope (see following section on pressors and inotropes). Do not use a pure vasopressor (e.g., phenylephrine).

If hypotension persists or is profound, norepinephrine may be implemented as single-agent therapy. Dobutamine may be added as an adjunct if response to norepinephrine is poor. In the case where hypotension is not present, then dobutamine is the initial form of pharmacological therapy as a single agent. If pharmacological BP support fails, then inotropic mechanical support such as intraaortic balloon pump is warranted.

In the case of acute VSD or MR, the mainstay therapy is dobutamine and nitroprusside first, deploying intraaortic balloon pump if these fail. Dobutamine improves contractility of the heart and decreases preload, while nitroprusside vasodilates promoting systemic blood flow. However, in MR the end goal therapy is surgical repair or replacement of the valve.

Medical Support: Pressors and Inotropes

Dopamine has dose-dependent effects. At rates 2.5 to 5 mcg/kg per minute, dopamine is alleged to have β1-adrenergic effects, delivering a chronotropic and inotropic effect on the heart. At 5 to 10 mcg/kg/min, dopamine is touted to have mixed α- and β1-adrenergic effect. At rates >10 mcg/kg per minute, α-adrenergic activity predominates, which increases SVR and BP. Initial loading doses are generally 2.5 to 5 mcg/kg per minute and titrate up to 20 to 50 mcg/kg per minute. Dopamine increases SVR, HR, and CO. Hypotension may occur if there is an imbalanced increase in SVR relative CO. The minimum dose of dopamine to achieve the desired effect is recommended to minimize arrhythmias, extremity gangrene, and ischemia.

Norepinephrine (NE) is also a first-line agent for BP support, enhancing both contractility and vasomotor tone. [9] NE is an α-adrenergic agonist and acts as a vasoconstrictor. Complications, similar to dopamine, are arrhythmias, extremity gangrene, and cardiac ischemia secondary to tachycardia. A starting dose of NE is 0.1 mcg/kg per minute, which can be titrated up to 2 mcg/kg per minute or an SBP >80 mm Hg.

Dobutamine, used when SBP is >90 mm Hg and signs of hypoperfusion exist, increases CO and lowers SVR and LV filling pressures, with minimum changes in BP. Dobutamine is a β1-adrenergic agonist with α- and β2-adrenergic effects. It increases myocardial contractility, improves coronary perfusion, and vasodilates peripheral vessels. It can be used in pure pump failure without hypotension or added after NE in those with hypotension to augment cardiac output. Starting doses are 2 to 5 mcg/kg per minute and titrated up to 20 mcg/kg per minute based on response. Arrhythmias, nausea, and headaches are potential complications.

Milrinone increases contractility, CO, and peripheral vasodilation. Its vasodilatory effects may exceed its inotropic effects, thus worsening hypotension. It is advised to have a pulmonary artery catheter in place to guide usage. Milrinone may be limited as monotherapy, although combination therapy may have more utility. The starting dose is 50 mcg/kg intravenously over 10 minutes, followed by a maintenance dose of 0.5 mcg/kg per minute.

Mechanical Support: Intraaortic Balloon Pump

An intra-aortic balloon pump (IABP) is a device placed in the aorta and timed to rapidly inflate on diastole and deflate on systole. It decreases afterload and myocardial work, thus decreasing myocardial oxygen consumption. Further, it improves coronary blood flow by increasing diastolic perfusion pressures and unloading of the LV. IABP should be considered in CS; however, IABP alone does not improve survival.

Revascularization Therapy

In AMI with CS, the most important lifesaving treatment is early revascularization (e.g., lytics, catheterization, or coronary artery bypass graft). Implementation of revascularization within 6 hours of diagnosing CS offers the best opportunity for survival, with the exception of those >75 years, who may have better survival with medical management alone.

Future Mechanical Management: Extracorporeal Membrane Oxygenation and Percutaneous Ventricular Assist Devices

The use of extracorporeal membrane oxygenation (ECMO) and percutaneous ventricular assist devices are options for CS patients who are refractory to IABP and inotropes. ECMO is a cardiopulmonary bypass method that provides oxygenation and biventricular support. Percutaneous ventricular assist devices unload the left ventricle and provide circulatory support, showing improvement of several hemodynamic parameters, including cardiac index, systolic and diastolic BP, and pulmonary arterial pressure, acting as a bridge to therapy or recovery.

Disposition and Discharge

Any patient with ongoing hypoxemia/positive pressure ventilation needs, evidence of CS, new cardiac ischemia, acute kidney injury (elevated BUN), or profound BNP elevation is at higher risk of short-term mortality and morbidity; these patients are best cared for in a more intensive care setting rather than a general medical floor. CS patients require intensive care unit admission at a site that can provide mechanical therapy if needed; this may require transfer.

Pearls of Care

1. ADHF can be hard to diagnose, and severe ADHF and CS require early management to improve survival.
2. Diagnosis of ADHF is based on history (known previous heart failure, dyspnea, orthopnea, PND, swelling), physical exam (vital signs, JVD, gallop, rales), and diagnostic tools (CXR, selective use of BNP, and echocardiogram if possible).
3. Stabilization in severe ADHF may require oxygen/ventilation support, diuresis or fluid therapy, inotropes and other vasoactive agents, or IABP.
4. The management goal is to remove or fix the precipitating factor while administering medical therapy based on the clinical presentation and the hemodynamics.
5. Disposition and discharge should follow a criterion that provides adequate monitoring and support, minimizes risk factors of mortality, and coincides with the patient's wishes.

References

1. Writing Group Members, Lloyd-Jones D, Adams RJ, et al. Heart disease and stroke statistics—2010 update: A report from the American Heart Association. *Circulation* 2010;121(7):e46–215.

2. Hochman JS, Buller CE, Sleeper LA. Cardiogenic shock complicating acute myocardial infarction—etiologies, management and outcome: a report from the SHOCK Trial Registry. Should we emergently revascularize Occluded Coronaries for cardiogenic shock? *J Am Coll Cardiol* 2000;36(3 Suppl A):1063–1070.

3. Goldberg RJ, Spencer FA, Szklo-Coxe M. Symptom presentation in patients hospitalized with acute heart failure. *Clin Cardiol* 2010;33(6):e73–e80.

4. McCullough PA, Nowak RM, McCord J. B-Type natriuretic peptide and clinical judgment in emergency diagnosis of heart failure: analysis from Breathing Not Properly (BNP) Multinational Study. *Circulation* 2002;106(4): 416–422.

5. Fonarow GC, Peacock WF, Phillips CO. Admission B-type natriuretic peptide levels and in-hospital mortality in acute decompensated heart failure. *J Am Coll Cardiol* 2007;49(19): 1943–1950.

6. Peacock WF, De Marco T, Fonarow GC. Cardiac troponin and outcome in acute heart failure. *N Engl J Med* 2008;358(20):2117–2126.

7. Nava S, Carbone G, DiBattista N. Noninvasive ventilation in cardiogenic pulmonary edema: a multicenter randomized trial. *Am J Respir Crit Care Med* 2003;168(12): 1432–1437.

8. Maisel AS, Peacock WF, McMullin N. Timing of immunoreactive B-type natriuretic peptide levels and treatment delay in acute decompensated heart failure: an ADHERE (Acute Decompensated Heart Failure National Registry) analysis. *J Am Coll Cardiol* 2008;52(7): 534–540.

9. De Backer D, Biston P, Devriendt J. Comparison of dopamine and norepinephrine in the treatment of shock. *N Engl J Med* 2010;362(9):779–789.

10. Fonarow GC, Adams KF, Jr., Abraham WT. Risk stratification for in-hospital mortality in acutely decompensated heart failure: classification and regression tree analysis. *JAMA* 2005;293(5): 572–580.

Chapter 5

Acute Myocardial Infarction, Acute Coronary Syndromes, Dysrhythmias, Pacemakers, and Automatic Implantable Cardioverter Defibrillators

Glen E. Michael and Robert E. O'Connor

Introduction

Acute coronary syndromes, dysrhythmias, and problems related to pacemakers and internal cardiac defibrillators are all frequently encountered in the emergency department (ED). Emergency providers should be skilled at identifying these conditions and be prepared to perform the critical interventions needed to stabilize stricken patients.

Acute myocardial ischemia includes unstable angina, non-ST-elevation myocardial infarction, and ST-elevation myocardial infarction. These syndromes require appropriate disposition and may require time-sensitive interventions to prevent death and disability.

Critically ill patients also present to the ED as a result of primary cardiac dysrhythmias, or they may develop dysrhythmias as a result of other life-threatening conditions, including acute ischemia. Emergency physicians must therefore be able to rapidly recognize and appropriately treat the wide array of cardiac dysrhythmias. Principles of recognition and management are easiest to remember when divided into the tachydysrhythmias (further separated into wide complex and narrow complex) and bradydysrhythmias.

The use of implantable cardiac defibrillators (ICDs) is growing at a tremendous rate, with over 150,000 implanted in 2003 compared to just over 20,000 in 1995.[1] Similar numbers of permanent pacemakers are placed each year in the United States.[2] Complications stemming from implantation and malfunction of these devices are not uncommon, and emergency physicians should be prepared to manage life-threatening conditions related to these devices.

Definition of Terms

Acute coronary syndrome (ACS): the clinical syndrome of acute myocardial ischemia ranging from unstable angina to myocardial infarction.

Bradydysrhythmias: disturbances in cardiac activity with rates less than 60 beats/min that compromise cardiac function.

Non-ST elevation myocardial infarction (NSTEMI): diagnosed by history, physical exam, elevated cardiac biomarkers, and a nondiagnostic electrocardiogram (ECG).

ST elevation myocardial infarction (STEMI): diagnosed by history, physical exam, and identification of ST-segment elevation on ECG.

Stable angina: due to a fixed stenosis of the coronary artery.

Tachydysrhythmias: electrical disturbances in cardiac activity with a rate over 100 beats/min that compromise cardiac function. The most unstable and immediately life-threatening tachydysrhythmias are ventricular in origin.

Unstable angina (UA): UA is usually diagnosed by history and exam alone, because biomarkers and ECGs are normal or nondiagnostic. UA is caused by transient platelet aggregation, coronary artery spasm, or coronary thrombosis. UA has at least one of the following: (1) occurs at rest or with minimal exertion and usually lasts longer than 20 minutes; (2) severe and described as chest discomfort of new onset; (3) occurs with a crescendo pattern that is more severe, prolonged, or increased in frequency compared to previously.[3]

Clinical Syndromes—Acute Coronary Syndrome and Myocardial Infarction

ACS is caused by an imbalance between myocardial oxygen supply and demand. The typical symptom of ACS is chest tightness that radiates to the left shoulder, left arm, left side of the lower jaw, and/or left side of the neck. This tightness is typically associated with diaphoresis, nausea and vomiting, and shortness of breath. Not all patients experience these "typical" symptoms and may instead complain of general malaise, palpitations, anxiety, or other vague, nonspecific complaints. The diagnostic utility of any specific combination of symptoms for ACS has poor predictive value. ACS does not include stable angina, which develops during a consistent level of exertion and resolves with rest.

When history and physical exam suggest ACS, stratification of patients is based on the interpretation of biomarkers and ECG findings (Fig. 5.1).[4] UA has biomarkers and ECGs that are normal or nondiagnostic. NSTEMI has elevated biomarkers with a nondiagnostic ECG. STEMI is recognized by ST-segment elevation on ECG regardless of biomarker levels.

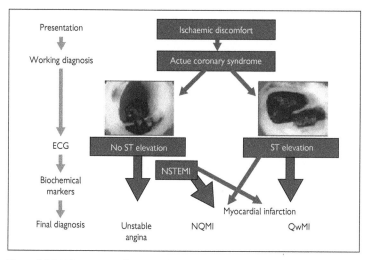

Figure 5.1 Initial assessment of patients admitted with suspected acute coronary syndrome. ECG, electrocardiogram; NSTEMI, non–ST elevation myocardial infarction.

Reproduced from Antman E. The re-emergence of anticoagulation in coronary disease. *Eur Heart J* 2004;6(B3).

General and Key Management Principles—Acute Coronary Syndromes

The ECG is a quick and reliable means to distinguish between the various causes of ACS, and it should be performed at the time of the first medical contact in patients suspected of having ACS. Early identification of STEMI is critical because immediate reperfusion therapy using angioplasty or fibrinolysis increases survival and functional recovery. When the first medical contact is in the prehospital setting, EMS personnel should obtain the initial ECG, which should then be interpreted immediately by qualified personnel either at the scene or via ECG transmission.[5] If the hospital emergency department is the site of first medical contact, an ECG should be obtained immediately on patient arrival. If the ECG shows a STEMI, reperfusion therapy is indicated either with fibrinolysis (time target is less than 30 minutes from first medical contact) or angioplasty (time target is less than 90 minutes from first medical contact). If the initial ECG does not demonstrate a STEMI, the patient could still have UA or NSTEMI, or he or she may not have ACS.

Ultrasensitive troponin I assays are the current state-of-the-art cardiac biomarkers for the risk stratification, diagnosis, and treatment of patients with suspected ACS.[6] Older biomarkers such as myoglobin and CK-MB have diminishing diagnostic utility. Nearly 80% of patients with AMI have an elevated troponin within 2 to 3 hours of emergency department presentation. Initial biomarkers may be normal or elevated in STEMI because ECG changes occur within minutes of arterial occlusion. To distinguish NSTEMI from UA, obtain serial troponins at baseline and 6–9 hours later.[3] Serial measurement of the ultrasensitive troponin assays may only require 4–6 hours to exclude NSTEMI. UA may turn out to be NSTEMI based on characteristic elevations in serum biomarkers, or it may evolve into a STEMI based on subsequent ECG tracings. Consequently, UA is treated the same as NSTEMI, until serial ECGs and biomarkers have excluded myocardial infarction.

Emergency Medical Systems for Acute Coronary Syndrome

It is imperative that individuals with symptoms suggestive of ACS call 911 immediately. The 911 call-taker can use an emergency medical dispatch (EMD) system to triage 911 calls for chest pain with very high sensitivity but very low specificity.[7] Calling 911 accomplishes several things: it begins the risk stratification process whereby the emergency medical service (EMS) call-taker assesses the patient using scripted questions, provides instructions for aspirin administration, instructs bystanders on the performance of CPR should the need arise, and mobilizes EMS providers. Unfortunately, many patients with ACS will call on friends or family for initial consultation, thus bypassing EMS dispatch. Whether public education campaigns on the need to call 911 will be more successful in the future remains to be determined.

EMS should develop ACS systems of care designed to reduce the time to reperfusion for STEMI patients given local resources. All EMS systems should have the capability to obtain prehospital ECGs to identify STEMI (and sometimes NSTEMI) shortly after first medical contact to allow for early direction of care. The ECG must be interpreted by someone qualified to identify STEMI whether that person is a paramedic at the scene, a physician at the hospital, or both. Many systems in the United States use paramedic ECG interpretation and have found it to be highly reliable.[8]

A number of successful models have been developed to minimize the time to reperfusion once a STEMI has been identified on ECG. Options include the following: prehospital fibrinolysis followed by transport to the hospital; transport to a non–percutaneous coronary intervention (PCI) hospital for in-hospital fibrinolysis; or transport to a PCI-capable center for PCI, which may include bypassing one or more non-PCI-capable centers. The 2010 American Heart Association Guidelines for Cardiopulmonary Resuscitation and Emergency Cardiovascular Care strongly recommend that systems which administer fibrinolytics in the prehospital setting include the following features: protocols using fibrinolytic checklists, 12-lead ECG acquisition and interpretation, experience in advanced life support, communication with the receiving institution, a medical director with training and experience in STEMI management, and continuous quality improvement.[9] Patients deemed ineligible for fibrinolytic therapy or who are in cardiogenic shock should be taken to a PCI-capable center (Fig. 5.2).[10]

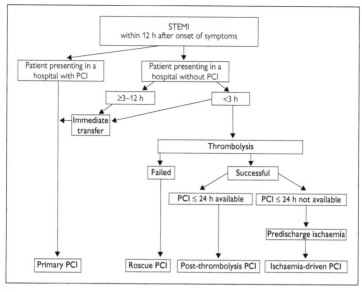

Figure 5.2 Flow chart of the treatment strategy for patients with acute ST elevation myocardial infarction (STEMI). PCI, percutaneous coronary intervention.

Reproduced from Elsasser A, Hamm C. Percutaneous coronary intervention guidelines: new aspects for the interventional treatment of acute coronary syndromes. *Eur Heart J* 2005;7(K7).

Reperfusion Therapy for STEMI

From time of first medical contact, fibrinolysis should ideally be initiated within 30 minutes, or PCI should be initiated within 90 minutes for patients with STEMI. It is reasonable to transport patients directly to the nearest PCI facility, bypassing closer EDs as necessary, in systems where time intervals between first medical contact and balloon times are less than 90 minutes and transport times are relatively short, in most case less than 30 minutes. Patients treated with fibrinolysis who have failed reperfusion as demonstrated by failure to resolve ECG findings should be transferred immediately for PCI. In addition, there is emerging evidence that patients treated with fibrinolysis who have resolution of ECG changes benefit from undergoing cardiac catheterization within 6 to 24 hours.[11]

Ruling Out Myocardial Infarction

Serial cardiac biomarkers are obtained for suspected ACS without diagnostic ECG. Elevated serum levels of troponin correlate with an increased risk of death, and greater elevations predict greater risk of adverse outcome. Serum levels of cardiac troponin require several hours to rise and thus may be normal during the initial hours of STEMI and NSTEMI. At least 4 to 6 hours are required to demonstrate or exclude NSTEMI. Rising cardiac troponin levels identify patients who might benefit from an early invasive strategy.[12]

When serial troponin levels are normal and ECG is nondiagnostic after 6 hours, patients are not having an NSTEMI and may be safely referred for provocative testing. Noninvasive tests for inducible myocardial ischemia (e.g., exercise or dobutamine stress tests) or anatomic evaluations of the coronary arteries (e.g., computed tomography [CT] angiography, cardiac magnetic resonance, myocardial perfusion imaging, or stress echocardiography) can distinguish patients requiring further treatment from those suitable for discharge from the ED.[13]

Ancillary Treatment for Acute Coronary Syndrome

Supplemental oxygen should be administered to patients with shortness of breath, congestive heart failure, or shock. Noninvasive monitoring of blood oxygen saturation can be used to determine the need for oxygen administration. An arterial oxyhemoglobin saturation <94% usually indicates a need for supplemental oxygen.[9]

Early administration of aspirin is recommended owing to its association with decreased mortality rates for ACS patients in several clinical trials. Multiple studies support the safety of aspirin administration. Unless the patient has a known aspirin allergy or active gastrointestinal hemorrhage, nonenteric aspirin should be given as soon as possible, either by bystanders, EMS personnel, or hospital personnel, to all patients with suspected ACS. It is reasonable to administer a 300-mg oral dose of clopidogrel to patients with suspected ACS (even without ECG or cardiac marker changes) who are unable to take aspirin because of hypersensitivity or major gastrointestinal intolerance.

Nitroglycerin has beneficial hemodynamic effects, including dilation of the coronary arteries (particularly in the region of plaque disruption), the peripheral arterial bed, and venous capacitance vessels. Patients with ischemic discomfort should receive up to three doses of sublingual or aerosol nitroglycerin at 3- to 5-minute intervals until pain is relieved or low blood pressure limits its use. Nitroglycerin should not be given to patients with suspected right ventricular infarct, which may be suspected on the basis of hypotension or bradycardia with clear lung fields. In such patients, a right-sided ECG should be obtained and may be helpful in identifying right ventricular infarcts.

Providers should administer analgesics, such as intravenous morphine, for chest discomfort unresponsive to nitrates. Although morphine is the preferred analgesic for patients with STEMI, other analgesics may be as effective but have not been used as extensively as morphine.

Patients with STEMI or moderate- to high-risk non-ST-segment elevation ACS should be given a loading dose of clopidogrel in addition to standard care (aspirin, anticoagulants, and reperfusion). Prasugrel (60 mg oral loading dose) may be substituted for clopidogrel in patients determined to have NSTEMI or STEMI prior to PCI.[14]

The use and efficacy of glycoprotein IIb/IIIa receptor inhibitors for treatment of patients with UA/NSTEMI have been well established. However, due to recent advances in interventional and conservative management of ACS, there is no current evidence supporting the routine use of GP IIb/IIIa inhibitor therapy prior to angiography in patients with STEMI.

Heparin is an indirect inhibitor of thrombin that has been widely used in ACS as adjunctive therapy for fibrinolysis and in combination with aspirin and other platelet inhibitors for the treatment of NSTEMI and UA. For in-hospital patients with NSTEMI managed with a planned initial conservative approach, fondaparinux, enoxaparin, or unfractionated heparin (UFH) may be used. For in-hospital patients with NSTEMI managed with a planned invasive approach, either enoxaparin or UFH may be used. For patients with STEMI managed with PCI or with fibrinolysis in the hospital or prehospital setting, either enoxaparin or UFH may be used.

For patients with ACS, there is no evidence to support the routine administration of IV beta-blockers in the prehospital setting or during initial assessment in the ED. IV beta-blocker therapy should only be used in specific situations such as severe hypertension or tachydysrhythmias. However, all patients with suspected ACS should have oral beta-blocker therapy initiated within the first 24 hours following symptom onset.[14] Administration of an oral ACE inhibitor is recommended within the first 24 hours after onset of symptoms in STEMI patients with pulmonary congestion or LV ejection fraction <40%, in the absence of hypotension. Many interventional cardiologists use statin pretreatment for patients who will be undergoing elective or urgent angioplasty in order to decrease the risk of periprocedural myocardial infarction.[15]

Clinical Syndromes—Wide Complex Tachycardia

The most unstable and immediately life-threatening tachydysrhythmias are those with wide QRS complexes (QRS duration greater than 120 msec). Ventricular fibrillation, ventricular tachycardia including torsades de pointes, and wide complex supraventricular tachycardias pose the greatest risk of decompensation.

Ventricular fibrillation (VF) is a grossly disorganized ventricular rhythm that accounts for many cases of sudden cardiac death. VF is uniformly fatal unless promptly recognized and treated.

Ventricular tachycardia (VT) is the most common cause of wide complex tachycardia.[16] VT is defined as any rhythm faster than 100 beats/min arising from below the AV node. VT is considered "nonsustained" when it spontaneously resolves within 30 seconds, whereas VT lasting longer than 30 seconds or requiring clinical intervention is considered "sustained." In *monomorphic VT* the morphology of QRS complexes is uniform throughout any given lead, while *polymorphic VT* displays continual variability in QRS morphology and axis within a given lead (Fig. 5.3).[17]

Torsades de pointes is a specific type of polymorphic VT in which the QRS complexes are characteristically seen to be "twisting" about the cardiac axis

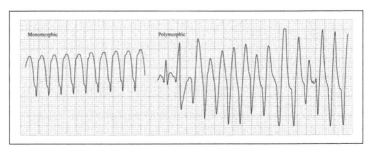

Figure 5.3 Examples of monomorphic and polymorphic ventricular tachycardia.

Reproduced from Edhouse J. Broad complex tachycardia—Part I. *BMJ* 2002;324(7339) with permission from BMJ Publishing Group Ltd.

(Fig. 5.4).[18] It is usually a result of QT prolongation, either due to congenital syndromes or secondary to medications, toxins, or metabolic abnormalities.

Supraventricular tachydysrhythmias with aberrant conduction or pre-excitation may also produce wide complex tachycardia. These can be difficult to distinguish from VT, but electrocardiographic clues can point to the diagnosis (Table 5.1). Adenosine can also be used to help differentiate between VT and wide complex SVT, but it should be used with extreme caution and never given in an irregular wide complex tachycardia, because it can convert SVT with pre-excitation into VF.

General and Key Management Principles—Wide Complex Tachycardia

Physicians tend to overdiagnose SVT with aberrancy and underdiagnose VT. When uncertain, all wide complex tachycardias should be treated as VT, which is far more common than SVT with aberrancy. Over 98% of patients presenting with a wide complex tachycardia that have a history of prior myocardial infarction or congestive heart failure will be in VT, not SVT.[16] Mistaking VT for SVT with aberrancy can have lethal consequences. In general, patients with SVT tend

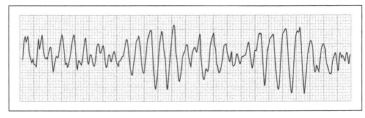

Figure 5.4 Torsades de pointes.

Reproduced from Edhouse J, Morris F. Broad complex tachycardia—Part II. *BMJ*. 2002;324(7340) with permission from BMJ Publishing Group Ltd.

Table 5.1 Differentiation between Ventricular Tachycardia and Supraventricular Tachycardia with Bundle Branch Block

If the tachycardia has a right bundle branch morphology (a predominantly positive QRS complex in lead V1), a ventricular origin is suggested if the following are present:

• QRS complex with duration >0.14 s

• Axis deviation

• A QS wave or predominantly negative complex in lead V6

• Concordance throughout the chest leads, with all deflections positive

• A single (R) or biphasic (QR or RS) R wave in lead V1

• A triphasic R wave in lead V1, with the initial R wave taller than the secondary R wave and an S wave that passes through the isoelectric line

If the tachycardia has a left bundle branch morphology (a predominantly negative deflection in lead V1), a ventricular origin is suggested if the following are present:

• Axis deviation

• QRS complexes with duration >0.16 s

• A QS or predominantly negative deflection in lead V6

• Concordance throughout the chest leads, with all deflections negative

• An rS complex in lead V1

Source: Reproduced from Edhouse J, Morris F. Broad complex tachycardia—Part II. *BMJ* 2002;324(7340) with permission from BMJ Publishing Group Ltd.

to be younger and tend not to have underlying coronary artery disease, whereas patients with VT tend to be older and have underlying structural heart disease.

Treatment of VF and pulseless VT includes providing high-quality CPR and cardiac defibrillation. The American Heart Association also recommends epinephrine 1 mg IV/IO every 3–5 minutes and amiodarone 300 mg IV/IO for VF or pulseless VT refractory to initial defibrillation attempts.[19]

For VT with pulses but instability evidenced by hypotension, altered mental status, ischemic chest pain, or other signs of end-organ dysfunction, immediate synchronized cardioversion at 100 joules should be performed. Synchronization may not be possible for polymorphic VT, in which case unsynchronized defibrillation may be required. For hemodynamically stable suspected VT, treatment should include an intravenous (IV) antiarrhythmic medication such as amiodarone (150 mg over 10 minutes, followed by a maintenance infusion of 1 mg/min for 6 hours) or procainamide (20–50 mg/min until arrhythmia corrected, QRS widens >50%, or hypotension develops, with a maximum dose of 17 mg/kg, followed by a maintenance infusion at 1–4 mg/min). If VT fails to respond to antiarrhythmic medication or instability ensues, synchronized cardioversion can be attempted.

Torsades de pointes is usually nonsustained, and its treatment requires addressing the underlying precipitant. Sustained torsades can be treated with cardioversion, but synchronization may not be possible and unsynchronized defibrillation may be required. Overdrive pacing at a rate over 120 beats/min and administration of IV magnesium sulfate are also effective at treating torsades de pointes.[20,21]

Adenosine can terminate a wide complex SVT but should be used with extreme caution for regular wide complex tachycardia and never given in an irregular wide complex tachycardia, because it can convert SVT with pre-excitation into VF.

Patients with wide complex tachycardias should generally be admitted from the ED to an inpatient critical care setting for further monitoring and evaluation

Clinical Syndromes—Narrow Complex Tachycardia

Narrow complex tachycardias tend to be more stable than their wide complex counterparts, but they may still cause significant hemodynamic compromise. Narrow complex tachycardias arise at or above the level of the atrioventricular node and include sinus tachycardia, atrial fibrillation, atrial flutter, atrioventricular nodal reentrant tachycardia, and atrioventricular reentrant tachycardia.

Sinus tachycardia is defined by a regular heart rate of greater than 100 beats per minute with consistent association between each normal P-wave and QRS complex. Sinus tachycardia is not a dysrhythmia, but its presence should prompt a search for other potentially life-threatening causes of the tachycardia.

Atrial fibrillation is the most common sustained dysrhythmia, with an overall prevalence of 1%–1.5%.[22] Atrial fibrillation is caused by multiple erratic foci of atrial depolarization, resulting in a fine, wavy ECG baseline and the absence of discernible P-waves. Conduction of these many atrial impulses across the AV node is variable and inconsistent, producing an irregular rhythm of QRS complexes (Fig. 5.5). The resultant heart rate varies depending on characteristics affecting the AV node such as beta-blocker use, but with normal AV conduction the rate is typically 100–180 beats/min. At high ventricular rates, atrial fibrillation can cause hypotension due to decreased diastolic filling time along with the loss of coordinated atrial contraction. Atrial fibrillation may be idiopathic, but it is frequently associated with an underlying physical stressor such as infection, cardiac ischemia, hypovolemia, or metabolic abnormality. In addition to directly managing the aberrant rhythm of atrial fibrillation, one should also consider possible underlying contributors to the dysrhythmia.

Atrial flutter produces characteristic broad, saw-toothed baseline waves with an atrial rate of about 300 beats/min (Fig. 5.6). In contrast to atrial fibrillation,

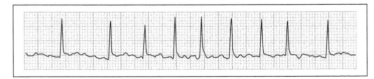

Figure 5.5 Atrial fibrillation.

Reproduced from Goodacre S, Irons R. Atrial arrhythmias. *BMJ* 2002;324(7337) with permission from BMJ Publishing Group Ltd.

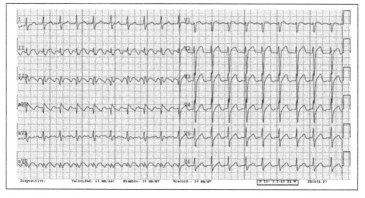

Figure 5.6 Atrial flutter. Arrows show characteristic saw-toothed flutter waves.

Reproduced from Stahmer SA, Cowan R. Tachydysrhythmias. *Emerg Med Clin North Am* 2006;24(1) with permission from Elsevier.

conduction across the AV node typically results in a regular ventricular rhythm. Most commonly, conduction across the AV node occurs in a 2:1 ratio, producing a ventricular rate of 150 beats/min, although 4:1 conduction and variable conduction are also common.[23] Similar to atrial fibrillation, the rapid ventricular rate and discordant atrial contraction of atrial flutter can result in hemodynamic compromise.

Atrioventricular reentrant tachycardia (AVRT) and *atrioventricular nodal reentrant tachycardia (AVNRT)* are both supraventricular tachycardias arising from the region of the AV junction. AVRT is most commonly associated with Wolff-Parkinson-White syndrome, while AVNRT is more common overall. AVRT and AVNRT occur when a reentrant loop circuit develops. In AVNRT, both the anterograde and retrograde limbs of the reentrant loop pass through the AV node. In AVRT, one limb passes through the AV node, while an accessory pathway exists between the atrium and ventricle outside of the AV node. Conduction in AVRT can be either orthodromic—passing anterograde through the AV node and then reentering the atria through the accessory pathway—or antidromic, passing first through the accessory pathway and then circling back to the atria through the AV node. Orthodromic AVRT results in a narrow QRS complex, while antidromic AVRT typically produces a wide QRS complex (Fig. 5.7).[24] Both AVNRT and orthodromic AVRT result in a regular rhythm, typically at a rate between 130 and 250 beats/min (Fig. 5.8).[23]

General and Key Management Principles— Narrow Complex Tachycardia

The treatment of sinus tachycardia should be aimed at the underlying condition precipitating the sinus tachycardia.

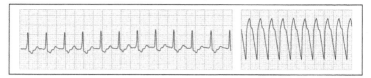

Figure 5.7 Orthodromic (*left*) and antidromic (*right*) atrioventricular reentrant tachycardia.

Reproduced from Esberger D, Jones S, Morris F. Junctional tachycardias. *BMJ* 2002;324(7338) with permission from BMJ Publishing Group Ltd

The management of other narrow complex tachycardias begins with assessing whether the patient is stable or unstable. Unstable patients, as evidenced by hypotension or signs of end-organ damage such as ischemic chest pain or altered mental status, should receive prompt synchronized cardioversion. For

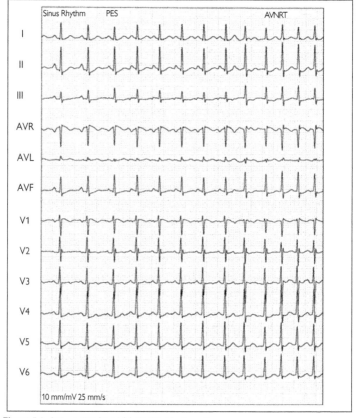

Figure 5.8 Atrioventricular nodal reentrant tachycardia.

Reproduced from Stahmer SA, Cowan R. Tachydysrhythmias. *Emerg Med Clin North Am* 2006;24(1) with permission from Elsevier.

regular narrow complex tachycardias such as atrial flutter the recommended initial cardioversion dose is 50–100 joules, while the recommended starting dose for irregular narrow complex rhythms (atrial fibrillation) is 120–200 joules.[19]

A more deliberate approach may be taken in stable patients, with the goal of identifying and treating the specific dysrhythmia present. Vagal maneuvers can be attempted while other treatment modalities are prepared. Adenosine may be given if narrow complex AVRT or AVNRT is suspected, as it successfully terminates these dysrhythmias in 95% of cases.[16] The treatment of stable atrial fibrillation or atrial flutter is typically aimed at rate control with beta-blockers (metoprolol 5 mg IV over 1–2 minutes) or calcium channel blockers (diltiazem 15–20 mg IV over 2 minutes). For patients with a known recent onset of stable atrial fibrillation or atrial flutter, conversion to sinus rhythm can be pursued via cardioversion or antiarrhythmic medication, though the optimal course of management and disposition of these patients is evolving.[25]

Clinical Syndromes—Bradydysrhythmias

Most cases of bradydysrhythmia are secondary to underlying medical conditions, with only about 15% being primarily attributable to an intrinsic defect in the cardiac conduction system (Table 5.2).[26] Bradydysrhythmias can be caused by sinoatrial (SA) dysfunction, such as sick sinus syndrome and sinus arrest, or by atrioventricular (AV) nodal dysfunction, such as first-, second-, and third-degree AV blocks.

Sinus bradycardia is often physiologic, and it is commonly seen in athletes, young healthy adults, and normal individuals during sleep. It is defined by an ECG revealing a heart rate less than 60 beats/min, consistent P waves 120–200 msec before each QRS complex, and a normal P wave axis. Pathologic sinus bradycardia is most often seen in acute inferior myocardial infarction but also occurs in sick sinus syndrome.

Table 5.2 Causes of Bradydysrhythmias	
Cause	Incidence (%)
Primary	15
Secondary	85
Acute coronary ischemia	40
Pharmacologic/toxicologic	20
Metabolic	5
Neurologic	5
Permanent pacemaker failure	2
Miscellaneous	13

Source: Reproduced from Brady WJ, Harrigan RA. Evaluation and management of bradyarrhythmias in the emergency department. *Emerg Med Clin North Am* 1998;16(2) with permission from Elsevier.

Sick sinus syndrome is a primary conduction disorder most commonly seen in elderly patients with idiopathic fibrosis of the SA node. It most commonly manifests as severe, persistent sinus bradycardia but may present in a variety of electrocardiographic ways, including periods of sinus arrest, SA block, junctional escape, tachy-brady syndrome, or intermittent atrial flutter or fibrillation.[27] *Tachy-brady syndrome* is characterized by paroxysmal episodes of atrial tachydysrhythmias interspersed with periods of atrial or ventricular bradycardia (Fig. 5.9).[28] *Sinoatrial block* occurs when an impulse generated by the SA node fails to conduct through the atrial myocardium, resulting in episodic pauses between P waves equal in duration to two or more P-P intervals. *Sinus arrest* is diagnosed when there is a prolonged pause without P wave activity, as a result of transient loss of SA node impulse formation. In contrast to SA block, there is no relationship between the length of the pause and the P-P interval in sinus arrest.

Atrioventricular nodal dysfunction is described as first, second, or third degree, corresponding to whether the dysfunction results in conduction delay, intermittent conduction blockade, or complete blockade. *First-degree AV block* is seen when the PR interval is constant and each P wave is reliably followed by a QRS complex, but the PR interval is greater than 200 msec (Fig. 5.10). First-degree AV block tends to be a stable rhythm, with a low risk of progression to complete heart block or life-threatening bradycardia.

Second-degree AV block occurs when atrial impulses are intermittently blocked from being conducted to the ventricles, resulting in some P waves that are not followed by a QRS complex. In the *Mobitz type I* (or "Wenckebach") form of second-degree block, conduction abnormalities at the AV node result in progressive lengthening of the PR interval ultimately leading to a P wave that is not followed by a QRS complex (Fig. 5.11). *Mobitz type II* also involves intermittent failure of conduction across the AV node, but unlike Mobitz type I the PR interval does not progressively lengthen and is constant (Fig. 5.12). The conduction

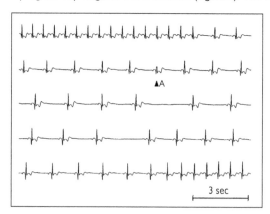

Figure 5.9 Tachy-brady syndrome.

Reproduced from Ufberg JW, Clark JS. Bradydysrhythmias and atrioventricular conduction blocks. *Emerg Med Clin North Am* 2006;24(1) with permission from Elsevier.

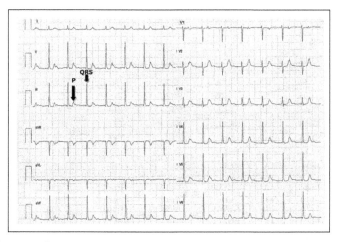

Figure 5.10 First-degree atrioventricular block.

Reproduced from Ufberg JW, Clark JS. Bradydysrhythmias and atrioventricular conduction blocks. *Emerg Med Clin North Am* 2006;24(1) with permission from Elsevier.

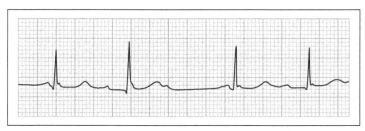

Figure 5.11 Second-degree atrioventricular block, Mobitz type I.

Reproduced from Da Costa D, Brady WJ, Edhouse J. Bradycardias and atrioventricular conduction block. *BMJ* 2002;324(7336) with permission from BMJ Publishing Group Ltd.

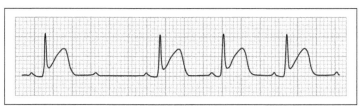

Figure 5.12 Second-degree atrioventricular block, Mobitz type II. Note the ST elevation here in lead II; this type of block can arise as a result of inferior myocardial infarction.

Reproduced from Da Costa D, Brady WJ, Edhouse J. Bradycardias and atrioventricular conduction block. *BMJ* 2002;324(7336) with permission from BMJ Publishing Group Ltd.

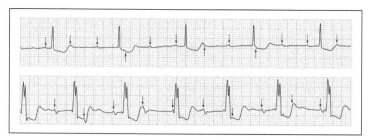

Figure 5.13 Third-degree atrioventricular block. Arrows show P waves, which are entirely independent of the QRS complexes. A pacemaker in the bundle of His produces a narrow QRS complex in the top figure, whereas more distal pacemakers tend to produce broader QRS complexes, as in the bottom figure.

Reproduced from Da Costa D, Brady WJ, Edhouse J. Bradycardias and atrioventricular conduction block. *BMJ*.2002;324(7336) with permission from BMJ Publishing Group Ltd.

abnormality in Mobitz type II usually occurs at the level of the bundle branches, and as a result most often leads to wide QRS complexes. Mobitz type I tends to be relatively stable, while Mobitz type II has a higher risk of progression to complete heart block.

Third-degree, or complete, AV block is defined by the complete dissociation of P waves and QRS complexes (Fig. 5.13). Atrial impulses are completely blocked from conducting through to the ventricles. Ventricular conduction depends upon a backup escape pacemaker, usually at a rate between 40 and 60 beats/min. QRS complexes remain narrow when driven by a junctional pacemaker within the AV node, but if the pacemaker is infranodal, then wide QRS complexes are produced, typically at a rate below 40 beats/min. Third-degree AV block is a highly unstable rhythm.

General and Key Management Principles—Bradydysrhythmias

The management of bradycardia depends upon the stability of the patient and his or her symptoms. In general, no acute intervention is needed in an asymptomatic patient with bradycardia, although a search for the underlying cause of the bradycardia should be initiated. Certain high-risk dysrhythmias such as third-degree AV block or Mobitz type II AV block still warrant close monitoring and cardiology consultation.

Transcutaneous cardiac pacing should immediately be considered in any unstable bradycardic patient who presents with hypotension, altered mental status, or other signs of end-organ compromise. Atropine 0.5 mg IV can be administered while preparing for transcutaneous pacing, but it is often ineffective for high-grade blocks.[19] Patients who respond to atropine may require a continuous infusion of epinephrine (2–10 mcg/min IV) or dopamine (2–10 mcg/kg per minute IV). Transcutaneous pacing should be initiated in patients who do not respond to atropine, and preparation for transvenous pacemaker placement should ensue.

Patients with symptomatic, but not unstable, bradycardia warrant close monitoring and may also benefit from medications such as atropine. Underlying causes of bradycardia must also be considered, including medication effects such as calcium channel blocker toxicity, metabolic abnormalities such as hypothyroidism, and cardiac ischemia.

Clinical Syndromes—Pacemaker and Implantable Cardiac Defibrillator Implantation Complications

ICDs and pacemakers are typically implanted in a subcutaneous pocket created in the subpectoral region. Leads that connect the device to the myocardium usually traverse the subclavian vein, and terminate at electrodes within the right atrium or right ventricle (Fig. 5.14). Complications of implantation of these devices may be related to the surgical creation of a device pocket, the transvenous approach to lead placement, or the interface between the myocardium and lead electrodes.[2]

Pocket complications include infection, hematoma formation, wound dehiscence, erosion, and device migration. *Pocket infection* may present on a spectrum from mild localized cellulitis to overwhelming sepsis. *Pocket hematoma* may develop shortly after implantation, and can lead to significant

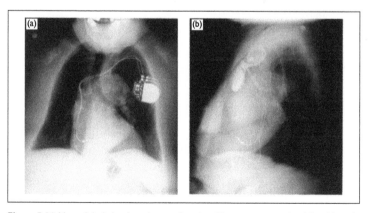

Figure 5.14 Normal dual-chambered pacemaker chest X-ray, posteroanterior (*a*) and lateral (*b*) views. The two leads of this dual-chambered pacemaker can be seen terminating in the right atrium and right ventricle.

Reproduced from Cardall TY, Chan TC, Brady WJ, et al. Permanent cardiac pacemakers: issues relevant to the emergency physician, Part I. *J Emerg Med* 1999;17(3) with permission from Elsevier.

bleeding or increase the risk of pocket infection. If the hematoma is palpable, it is likely large enough to require treatment. *Wound dehiscence* and *pocket erosion* are not usually life-threatening but do increase the risk of pocket infection. Wound dehiscence is usually an early complication occurring within days of implantation, while erosion may occur years after placement. *Device migration* is usually a chronic complication, resulting from gradual movement of the device away from the implantation site to surrounding tissue.

Lead placement complications include lead infection, pneumothorax, hemothorax, and venous thrombosis. *Lead infection* is rare, but has an extremely high risk of mortality. Presenting signs and symptoms often include fevers, chills, and pulmonary involvement. *Pneumothorax* or *hemothorax* may occur following implantation as a result of the subclavian approach to lead placement. The overall incidence of pneumothorax following pacemaker placement is under 2%, with about half of these requiring intervention.[29] *Venous thrombosis* related to transvenous lead placement may occur acutely or chronically. Acute thrombosis usually presents with pain or swelling of the ipsilateral arm, and the diagnosis is confirmed by duplex ultrasonography.

Electrode-myocardium interface complications include *electrode dislodgement* and *lead penetration*.[2,30] Dislodgement of the electrode from the myocardium may result in lead migration (Fig. 5.15), which can cause pacemaker

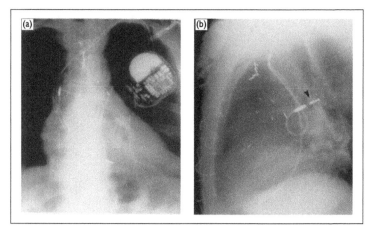

Figure 5.15 Lead dislodgement and migration seen on posteroanterior (*a*) and lateral (*b*) views of the chest. In these films, a dual-chambered pacemaker is seen with dislodgement of both leads. The atrial lead and the tip migrated to the azygos vein through the superior vena cava (arrow). The ventricular lead has dislodged from the ventricular wall but is still in the right ventricle.

Reproduced from Cardall TY, Chan TC, Brady WJ, et al. Permanent cardiac pacemakers: issues relevant to the emergency physician, Part I. *J Emerg Med* 1999;17(3) with permission from Elsevier.

malfunction, thrombosis formation, or life-threatening dysrhythmias when the electrode makes contact with other areas of the myocardium. Penetration of a lead through the myocardium is usually an acute complication of lead placement. However, recognition may be delayed and as a result patients may present to the ED after pacemaker or ICD implantation with pericarditis, pericardial effusion, or pericardial tamponade. Diagnosis of this complication is facilitated by bedside transthoracic ultrasound.

General and Key Management Principles— Pacemaker and Implantable Cardiac Defibrillator Implantation Complications

Any suspected pocket infection should be considered life-threatening and should be treated aggressively. Definitive treatment requires removal of the device. The role of the emergency physician is to obtain appropriate cultures, initiate antibiotic therapy with MRSA coverage, order chest radiographs, and arrange admission to the appropriate surgical service.[2] Treatment of a pocket hematoma often requires surgical exploration; needle aspiration in the ED is not recommended. Treatment of both dehiscence and erosion involves surgical debridement. No treatment for device migration is necessary unless the migration results in device malfunction, infection, or risk of erosion.

ED management of lead infection is similar to that for pocket infection, and admission for definitive management, including urgent lead removal, is required. Treatment of venous thrombosis related to lead placement involves anticoagulation and is similar to other forms of venous thrombosis. Pneumothroax and hemothorax related to lead placement are treated just as when these complications occur after other central lines.

Electrode displacement resulting in dysrhythmia may require acute treatment of the dysrhythmia, including placement of alternative temporary pacing. Lead penetration through myocardium resulting in percardial tamponade may require emergent pericardiocentesis.

Clinical Syndromes—Pacemaker and Implantable Cardiac Defibrillator Malfunction

Abnormalities of pacemaker function include failure to pace, failure to capture, undersensing, and pacemaker-induced dysrhythmias. Failure to pace occurs when a pacemaker fails to deliver an impulse when pacing should occur, and it may be due to oversensing, lead malfunction, battery failure, or electromagnetic interference.[30] Oversensing is caused by the pacemaker detecting an electrical signal, such as skeletal muscle myopotentials, that it inappropriately interprets as normal cardiac activity. As a result, the pacemaker inappropriately inhibits impulse generation. Other causes of failure to pace include battery failure or lead malfunction.

Failure to capture occurs when the pacemaker attempts to generate a stimulus as evidenced by the presence of a pacing artifact on ECG but fails to induce cardiac depolarization. This may be caused by lead damage, battery weakness, cardiac ischemia, myocardial refractoriness due to medications or metabolic abnormalities, or an increase in the voltage threshold needed at the electrode-myocardium interface to trigger depolarization. The latter condition is referred to as "exit block," and it is most commonly seen in the first month after implantation as a result of fibrosis and scarring of the myocardial tissue at the electrode interface.

Undersensing occurs when the pacemaker fails to detect native cardiac activity. This can result in inappropriate pacing over a normal cardiac rhythm. Undersensing may be caused by mechanical lead problems or by a change in the native cardiac rhythm such as a loss of amplitude, PVCs, new bundle branch block, or atrial fibrillation.

Pacemaker-mediated dysrhythmias include pacemaker-mediated tachycardia, runaway pacemaker, and dysrhythmias caused by lead dislodgement. *Pacemaker-mediated tachycardia* occurs in dual-chamber pacemakers with atrial sensing. This condition is usually precipitated by a PVC. The PVC causes a retrograde P wave, which is inappropriately sensed as normal atrial activity by the pacemaker. In response to atrial sensing, the pacemaker triggers a ventricular stimulus, which in turn produces another retrograde P wave, and a reentrant tachycardia ensues (Fig. 5.16).[31] Primary component failure can result in *runaway pacemaker*, in which the pacemaker inappropriately rapidly delivers

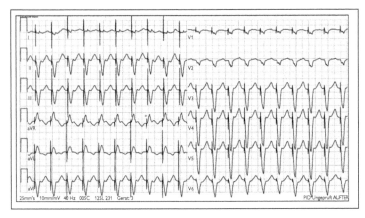

Figure 5.16 Pacemaker-mediated tachycardia. A broad complex tachycardia with pacing spikes (arrows) preceding each broad complex beat.

Reproduced from Ullah W, Stewart A. Pacemaker-mediated tachycardia. *Heart* 2010;96(13) with permission from BMJ Publishing Group Ltd.

stimuli at rates up to 400 impulses per minute. This can induce ventricular tachycardia or fibrillation. Dysrhythmias can also be caused by *lead dislodgement*, as a lead tip bouncing against the ventricular wall can induce ventricular tachycardia or fibrillation.

ICDs are susceptible to most of the same malfunctions seen in pacemakers. Unsuccessful defibrillation or failure to sense by an ICD may result in a sustained dysrhythmia and cardiac arrest. Patients often present to the ED after ICD shock delivery. After any ICD firing the patient should be monitored in the ED while awaiting cardiology consultation and device interrogation. Cardiac monitoring, a thorough history and examination, ECG, laboratory studies, and chest radiography should be performed to determine whether the ICD shocks were appropriate and whether there was any underlying pathology leading to the shock.

General and Key Management Principles—Pacemaker and Implantable Cardiac Defibrillator Malfunction

Oversensing can be corrected by application of a magnet, which causes most pacemakers to revert to a default mode of asynchronous pacing. When the magnet is applied, the pacemaker's sensing function is turned off, and the pacemaker automatically delivers impulses at a default rate.

Failure to pace from battery failure or lead malfunction requires treatment of the underlying dysrhythmia and may necessitate temporary external pacing in the ED. Failure to capture may be corrected by adjusting the pacemaker's voltage settings, but it may require transient transcutaneous pacing in the ED until the device can be interrogated and reprogrammed.

Pacemaker-mediated tachycardia is usually aborted by applying a magnet to the pacemaker, although adenosine may also be effective if a magnet is unavailable or unsuccessful. Magnet application may slow a runaway pacemaker, but surgical disconnection of the pacemaker leads is sometimes required for definitive treatment. Treatment of dysrhythmias caused by lead dislodgement involves managing the resultant dysrhythmia in a standard fashion and removing or repositioning the dislodged lead.

Patients experiencing recurrent inappropriate ICD shocks, which can occur as a result of sensing malfunction or increased frequency of NSVT, may need to have their device temporarily deactivated. In most modern ICDs this can be accomplished by placing a magnet over the ICD generator.

Management of cardiac arrest in patients with ICDs or pacemakers is for the most part similar to other patients, and standard ACLS guidelines apply. One caveat is external defibrillation, as externally defibrillating directly over a pacemaker or ICD has a high likelihood of damaging the implanted device. Defibrillation pads should be placed away from the pacemaker or ICD generator if possible. This is best achieved by placing the pads or paddles in an anterior-posterior configuration. In pacemaker-dependent patients, be prepared to provide external pacing after defibrillation due to the potential for pacemaker damage.

General and Key Management Controversies

The diagnosis of ACS is a dynamic process involving clinical identification of key elements from the history and physical exam, in conjunction with identification of abnormal biomarkers and ECG tracings. Treatment of ACS is directed at rapid identification of STEMI with early reperfusion using fibrinolysis or angioplasty. Identification of NSTEMI requires identification of an underlying cause and usually requires cardiac catheterization on an urgent basis. Correct identification and treatment of dysrhythmias is an essential skill in emergency medicine and may be life saving. Patients with pacemakers and automatic implantable cardioverter defibrillators (AICDs) will present to the ED when they are experiencing problems, and emergency physicians should be capable of identifying and treating emergent complications from these devices.

Pearls of Care

1. Patients suspected of having ACS should have an ECG performed at the time of first medical contact.
2. Patients with STEMI should receive rapid reperfusion.
3. Patients suspected of having ACS should have serial biomarkers obtained, especially if the initial ECG is not diagnostic for STEMI.
4. Patients with dysrhythmias should be assessed and treated emergently if rate-dependent hypoperfusion is suspected.
5. Emergency physicians should be facile in the identification and treatment of pacemaker and AICD-related malfunctions.

References

1. Jauhar S, Slotwiner DJ. The economics of ICDs. *N Engl J Med* 2004;351(24): 2542–2544.

2. Cardall TY, Chan TC, Brady WJ, et al. Permanent cardiac pacemakers: issues relevant to the emergency physician, Part I. *J Emerg Med* 1999;17(3):479–489.

3. Anderson JL, Adams CD, Antman EM, et al. ACC/AHA 2007 guidelines for the management of patients with unstable angina/non ST-elevation myocardial infarction: a report of the American College of Cardiology/American Heart Association Task Force on Practice Guidelines (Writing Committee to Revise the 2002 Guidelines for

the Management of Patients With Unstable Angina/Non ST-Elevation Myocardial Infarction): developed in collaboration with the American College of Emergency Physicians, the Society for Cardiovascular Angiography and Interventions, and the Society of Thoracic Surgeons: endorsed by the American Association of Cardiovascular and Pulmonary Rehabilitation and the Society for Academic Emergency Medicine. *Circulation* 2007;116(7):e148–e304.

4. Antman E. The re-emergence of anticoagulation in coronary disease. *Euro Heart J Suppl* 2004;6:B2–B8.

5. Ting HH, Krumholz HM, Bradley EH, et al. Implementation and integration of pre-hospital ECGs into systems of care for acute coronary syndrome: a scientific statement from the American Heart Association Interdisciplinary Council on Quality of Care and Outcomes Research, Emergency Cardiovascular Care Committee, Council on Cardiovascular Nursing, and Council on Clinical Cardiology. *Circulation* 2008;118(10):1066–1079.

6. Casals G, Filella X, Augé JM, Bedini JL. Impact of ultrasensitive cardiac troponin I dynamic changes in the new universal definition of myocardial infarction. *Am J Clin Pathol* 2008;130(6):964–968.

7. Sporer KA, Youngblood GM, Rodriguez RM. The ability of emergency medical dispatch codes of medical complaints to predict ALS prehospital interventions. *Prehosp Emerg Care* 2007;11(2):192–198.

8. Le May MR, Dionne R, Maloney J, et al. Diagnostic performance and potential clinical impact of advanced care paramedic interpretation of ST-segment elevation myocardial infarction in the field. *CJEM* 2006;8(6):401–407.

9. O'Connor RE, Bossaert L, Arntz HR, et al. Part 9: acute coronary syndromes: 2010 International Consensus on Cardiopulmonary Resuscitation and Emergency Cardiovascular Care Science with Treatment Recommendations. *Circulation* 2010;122(16 Suppl 2):S422–S465.

10. Elsasser A. Percutaneous coronary intervention guidelines: new aspects for the interventional treatment of acute coronary syndromes. *Euro Heart J Suppl* 2005;7(Suppl K):K5–K9.

11. Cantor WJ, Fitchett D, Borgundvaag B, et al. Routine early angioplasty after fibrinolysis for acute myocardial infarction. *N Engl J Med* 2009;360(26):2705–2718.

12. Narain VS, Gupta N, Sethi R, et al. Clinical correlation of multiple biomarkers for risk assessment in patients with acute coronary syndrome. *Indian Heart J* 2008;60(6):536–542.

13. Madsen T, Mallin M, Bledsoe J, et al. Utility of the emergency department observation unit in ensuring stress testing in low-risk chest pain patients. *Crit Pathw Cardiol* 2009;8(3):122–124.

14. O'Connor RE, Brady W, Brooks SC, et al. Part 10: acute coronary syndromes: 2010 American Heart Association Guidelines for Cardiopulmonary Resuscitation and Emergency Cardiovascular Care. *Circulation* 2010;122(18 Suppl 3):S787–S817.

15. Patti G, Chello M, Gatto L, et al. Short-term atorvastatin preload reduces levels of adhesion molecules in patients with acute coronary syndrome undergoing percutaneous coronary intervention. Results from the ARMYDA-ACS CAMs (Atorvastatin for Reduction of MYocardial Damage during Angioplasty-Cell Adhesion Molecules) substudy. *J Cardiovasc Med (Hagerstown)* 2010;11(11):795–800.

16. Shah CP, Thakur RK, Xie B, Hoon VK. *Clinical approach to wide QRS complex tachycardias. Emerg Med Clin North Am* 1998;16(2):331–360.

17. Edhouse J, Morris F. Broad complex tachycardia—Part II. *BMJ* 2002; 324(7340):776–779.

18. Edhouse J. Broad complex tachycardia—Part I. *BMJ* 2002;324(7339):719–722.

19. Neumar RW, Otto CW, Link MS, et al. Part 8: Adult advanced cardiovascular life support: 2010 American Heart Association Guidelines for Cardiopulmonary Resuscitation and Emergency Cardiovascular Care. *Circulation* 2010;122(18 Suppl 3):S729–S767.

20. Tzivoni D, Banai S, Schuger C, et al. Treatment of torsade de pointes with magnesium sulfate. *Circulation* 1988;77(2):392–397.

21. Vukmir RB. Torsades de Pointes: a review. *Am J Emerg Med* 1991;9(3):250–255.

22. Goodacre S, Irons R. Atrial arrhythmias. *BMJ* 2002;324(7337):594–597.

23. Stahmer SA, Cowan R. Tachydysrhythmias. *Emerg Med Clin North Am* 2006;24(1):11–40, v–vi.

24. Esberger D, Jones S, Morris F. Junctional tachycardias. *BMJ* 2002;324(7338):662–665.

25. Stiell IG, Clement CM, Brison RJ, et al. Variation in management of recent-onset atrial fibrillation and flutter among academic hospital emergency departments. *Ann Emerg Med* 2011;57(1):13–21.

26. Brady WJ, Harrigan RA. Evaluation and management of bradyarrhythmias in the emergency department. *Emerg Med Clin North Am* 1998;16(2):361–388.

27. Da Costa D, Brady WJ, Edhouse J. Bradycardias and atrioventricular conduction block. *BMJ* 2002;324(7336):535–538.

28. Ufberg JW, Clark JS. Bradydysrhythmias and atrioventricular conduction blocks. *Emerg Med Clin North Am* 2006;24(1):1–9, v.

29. Aggarwal RK, Connelly DT, Ray SG, 30. Ball J, Charles RG. Early complications of permanent pacemaker implantation: no difference between dual and single chamber systems. *Br Heart J* 1995;73(6):571–575.

30. Chan TC, Cardall TY. Electronic pacemakers. *Emerg Med Clin North Am* 2006;24(1):179–194, vii.

31. Ullah W, Stewart A. Pacemaker-mediated tachycardia. *Heart* 2010;96(13):1062.

Chapter 6

Acute Kidney Injury in the Emergency Department

John A. Kellum

Introduction

The terms *acute kidney injury (AKI)* and *acute renal failure* are not synonymous. While the term *renal failure* is best reserved for patients who have lost renal function to the point that life can no longer be sustained without intervention, *AKI* is used to describe patients with earlier or milder forms of acute renal dysfunction as well as those with overt failure. Although the analogy is imperfect, the AKI–renal failure relationship can be thought of as being similar to acute coronary syndrome and ischemic heart failure. AKI is intended to describe the entire spectrum of disease from relatively mild to severe. By contrast, renal failure is defined as renal function inadequate to clear the waste products of metabolism despite the absence of or correction of hemodynamic or mechanical causes. Clinical manifestations of renal failure (either acute or chronic) include the following:

- Uremic symptoms (drowsiness, nausea, hiccough, twitching)
- Hyperkalemia
- Hyponatremia
- Metabolic acidosis

Conversely, clinical manifestations of AKI can be mild or even absent, especially early in the course of the disease.

Diagnosis and Classification of Acute Kidney Injury

International consensus criteria for AKI have been developed. The acronym RIFLE is used to describe three levels of renal impairment (risk, injury, and failure) and two clinical outcomes (loss and end-stage kidney disease) (Fig. 6.1).

The RIFLE classification system includes separate criteria for serum creatinine and urine output. If a patient has criteria for multiple RIFLE categories, the patient is placed in the worst category for which they have criteria. Note that

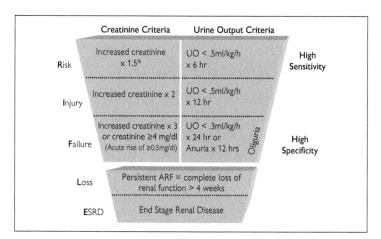

Figure 6.1 RIFLE.

*Recently "risk" was expanded by the Acute Kidney Injury Network to include any increase in serum creatinine of at least 0.3 mg/dL, even if less than 50% increase, as long as it is documented to occur over 48 hr or less. ARF, acute renal failure; ESRD, end-stage renal disease; UO, urine output.

RIFLE-F is present even if the increase in SCrt is <3-fold so long as the new SCrt is ≥4.0 mg/dL in the setting of an acute increase of at least 0.5 mg/dL. The shape the figure denotes the fact that more patients (high sensitivity) will be included in the mild category, including some without actually having renal failure (less specificity). In contrast, at the bottom, the criteria are strict and therefore specific, but some patients will be missed.

Oliguria

Persistent oliguria may be a feature of acute renal failure, but nonoliguric renal failure also occurs. Patients may continue to make urine despite an inadequate glomerular filtration. Although prognosis is often better if urine output is maintained, use of diuretics to promote urine output does not seem to improve outcome (and some studies even suggest harm).

Incidence and Progression

AKI occurs in 35%–65% of intensive care unit (ICU) admissions and 5%–20% of general hospital admissions. Mortality rates increase significantly with AKI and most studies show a 3- to 5-fold increase in the risk of death in hospital with AKI compared to patients without AKI. Furthermore, increases in severity of AKI are associated with a stepwise increase in risk of death such that patients reaching RIFLE-F are far more likely to die prior to hospital discharge compared to patients who do not progress from RIFLE-R or RIFLE-I. Hospital mortality rates for ICU patients with AKI are approximately as follows: R, 9%; I, 11%; and F, 26%, compared to 6% for ICU patients without AKI. Unfortunately, more than 50% of patients with RIFLE-R progress to class I (in approximately 1–2 days) or F (in approximately 3–4 days) and almost 30% of RIFLE-I progress to F.

Risk Factors for Acute Kidney Injury

Risk factors for developing AKI as defined by RIFLE criteria:
- Sepsis
- Increasing age, especially age >62 years
- Race; Black patients are more likely to develop RIFLE-F
- Greater severity of illness as per APACHE III or SOFA scores
- Preexisting chronic kidney disease
- Prior admission to a non–ICU ward in the hospital
- Surgical admissions more likely than medical admissions
- Cardiovascular disease
- Emergent surgeries
- Patients on mechanical ventilators

Etiology of Acute Kidney Injury

Clinical features may suggest the cause of AKI and dictate further investigation. AKI is common in the critically ill, especially in patients with sepsis and other forms of systemic inflammation (e.g., major surgery, trauma, burns), but other causes must be considered. In sepsis, the kidney often has a normal histological appearance.

Volume-Responsive Acute Kidney Injury
It is estimated that as many as 50% of cases of AKI are "fluid responsive," and the first step in managing any case of AKI is to ensure appropriate fluid resuscitation. However, volume overload is a key factor contributing to the mortality attributable to AKI, so ongoing fluid administration to non-fluid-responsive patients should be discouraged. In general, fluid resuscitation should be guided by hemodynamic monitoring.

Sepsis-Induced Acute Kidney Injury
Sepsis is a primary cause or contributing factor in more than 50% of cases of AKI, including those cases severe enough to require renal replacement therapy (RRT). Patients with sepsis develop AKI at rates as high as 40% even when considering patients outside the ICU. Septic shock appears to be an important factor in the development of sepsis-induced AKI; however, patients without overt shock do not appear to be any less likely to develop AKI.

Hypotension

Hypotension is an important risk factor for AKI; many patients with AKI have experienced at least one episode of hypotension. Treating fluid-responsive AKI with fluid resuscitation is clearly an important step, but many patients will also require vasoactive therapy (e.g., dopamine, norepinephrine) to maintain arterial blood pressure. Despite a common belief among many practitioners, norepinephrine does not increase the risk of AKI compared to dopamine, and in animals with sepsis, renal blood flow actually increases with norepinephrine.

Postoperative Acute Kidney Injury

Risk factors include hypovolemia, hypotension, major abdominal surgery, and sepsis. Surgical procedures (particularly gynecological) may be complicated by damage to the lower urinary tract with an obstructive nephropathy. Abdominal aortic aneurysm surgery may be associated with renal artery disruption. Cardiac surgery may be associated with atheroembolism and sustained periods of reduced arterial pressure as well as systemic inflammation.

Other Causes

Nephrotoxins may cause renal failure via direct tubular injury, interstitial nephritis, or renal tubular obstruction. In patients with AKI, all nephrotoxins that can be stopped should be.

Rhabdomyolysis is suggested by myoglobinuria and raised creatine kinase in patients who have suffered crush injury, limb ischemia, coma, or prolonged seizures.

Glomerular disease is suggested by red cell casts, hematuria, proteinuria, and systemic features (e.g., hypertension, purpura, arthralgia, vasculitis). Renal biopsy or specific blood tests (e.g., Goodpasture's syndrome, vasculitis) are required to confirm diagnosis and guide appropriate treatment.

Hemolytic uremic syndrome is suggested by hemolysis, uremia, thrombocytopenia, and neurological abnormalities.

Crystal nephropathy is suggested by the presence of crystals in the urinary sediment. Microscopic examination of the crystals confirms the diagnosis (e.g., urate, oxalate). Release of purines and urate is responsible for acute renal failure in the tumor lysis syndrome.

In renovascular disorders loss of vascular supply may be diagnosed by renography. Complete loss of arterial supply may occur in abdominal trauma or aortic disease (particularly dissection). More commonly, the arterial supply is partially compromised (e.g., renal artery stenosis) and blood flow is further reduced by hemodynamic instability or locally via drug therapy (e.g., nonsteroidal anti-inflammatory drugs [NSAIDs], ACE inhibitors). Renal vein obstruction may be due to thrombosis or external compression (e.g., raised intra-abdominal pressure).

Abdominal compartment syndrome is suggested by oliguria, a firm abdomen on physical examination, and increased airway pressures (secondary to upward pressure on the diaphragm). Diagnosis is likely when sustained increased intra-abdominal pressures (bladder pressure measured at end expiration in the supine position) exceed 25 mm Hg. However, abdominal compartment syndrome may occur with intra-abdominal pressures as low as 10 mm Hg. Surgical decompression is often required, and early surgical consultation is advisable.

Nephrotoxins

The following are some common nephrotoxins:

- Allopurinol
- Organic solvents
- Aminoglycosides
- Paraquat
- Amphotericin
- Pentamidine
- Furosemide
- IV radiographic contrast
- Herbal medicines
- Sulphonamides
- Heavy metals
- Thiazides
- NSAIDs

Clinical Consequences of Acute Kidney Injury

Until recently it was assumed that patients with AKI died not because of AKI itself but secondary to their underlying disease. Several studies, however, have documented a substantial mortality attributable to AKI after controlling for other variables, including chronic illness and underlying severity of acute illness. Table 6.1 lists some of the more important clinical consequences of AKI.

Management

The management of AKI in the emergency department involves simultaneous general support and workup for the cause of AKI. Identification and correction of reversible causes of AKI are critical. All cases require careful attention to fluid management and nutritional support.

General Measures

Close monitoring of urine output and serum creatinine is required. While it may take 24–48 hours for AKI to manifest, early changes in serum creatinine may be detectable within a few hours and changes in urine output (if they occur) may be noted even earlier. New biomarkers such as neutrophil gelatinase associated lipocalin (NGAL) may be detectable even earlier in the course of AKI. Once AKI is suspected, obstruction or hypovolemia should be excluded. Renal ultrasound

Table 6.1 Clinical Consequences of Acute Kidney Injury

System	Mechanisms	Complications
Electrolyte disturbances	Hyponatremia Hyperkalemia	CNS (see below)
		Malignant arrhythmias
Acid-base (decreased chloride excretion, accumulation of organic anions like PO_4, decreased albumin→ decreased buffering)	1) Down-regulation of beta-receptors, increased iNOS) 2) Hyperchloremia 3) Impairing the insulin resistance 4) Innate immunity	1) Decreased cardiac output, blood pressure 2) Lung, intestinal injury, decreases gut barrier function 3) Hyperglycemia. Increased protein breakdown 4) See below
Cardiovascular	Volume overload	Congestive heart failure
		Secondary hypertension
Pulmonary	1) Volume overload, decreased oncotic pressure 2) Infiltration and activation of lung neutrophils by cytokines 3) Uremia	1) Pulmonary edema, pleural effusions 2) Acute lung injury 3) Pulmonary hemorrhage
Gastrointestinal	1) Volume overload 2) Gut ischemia and reperfusion injury	1) Abdominal compartment syndrome 2) Acute gastric and duodenal ulcer→ bleeding; impaired nutrient absorption
Immune	1) Tissue edema 2) Decreased clearance of oxygen free radicals 3) White cell dysfunction	1) Increased risk of infection 2) Delayed wound healing
Hematological	1) Decreased synthesis of red blood cells; increased destruction of red blood cells, blood loss 2) Decreased production of erythropoietin, von Willebrand's factor	1) Anemia 2) Bleeding
Nervous system	1) Secondary hepatic failure, malnutrition, altered drug metabolism 2) Hyponatremia, acidosis 3) Uremia	1) Altered mental status 2) Seizures, impaired consciousness, coma 3) Myopathy, neuropathy→ prolonged length on mechanical ventilation
Pharmacokinetics and dynamics	Increased volume of distribution, decreased availability, albumin binding, elimination	Drug toxicity or underdosing

can be helpful in ruling out hypdronephrosis and also provides a measure of kidney size, which can be helpful in detecting chronic kidney disease (e.g., small kidneys).

Urinary Tract Obstruction

Lower tract obstruction requires the insertion of a catheter (suprapubic if there is urethral disruption) to allow decompression. Ureteric obstruction requires urinary tract decompression by nephrostomy or stent. A massive diuresis is common after decompression, so it is important to ensure adequate circulating volume to prevent secondary AKI.

Hemodynamic Management

Fluid-responsive AKI may be reversible in its early stage. Careful fluid management to ensure adequate circulating volume and any necessary inotrope or vasopressor support to ensure renal perfusion will help improve chances for renal recovery. Admission to intensive care and use of hemodynamic monitoring should be considered for all patients with AKI and is mandatory for patients not responding to conservative therapy.

Glomerular Disease

Fewer than 1% of patient presenting with AKI will have glomerular disease. A history of renal disease or vasculitis should increase suspicion. Red blood cell casts in the urine are almost diagnostic. Specific therapy in the form of immunosuppressive drugs may be useful after diagnosis has been confirmed.

Interstitial Nephritis

Acute interstitial nephritis most often results from drug therapy. However, other causes include autoimmune disease and infection (e.g., Legionella, leptospirosis, streptococcus, cytomegalovirus). Numerous drugs have been implicated, but the most common are:

- Antibiotics (penicillins, cephalosporins, sulfa, rifampin, quinilones)
- Diuretics (furosemide, bumetanide, thiazides)
- NSAIDs (including selective COX-2 inhibitors)
- Allopurinol
- Cimetidine (rarely other H-2 blockers)
- Proton pump inhibitors (omeprazole, lansoprazole)
- Indinavir
- 5-aminosalicylates

Urine sediment usually reveals white cells, red cells, and white cell casts. Eosinophiluria is present in about two-thirds of cases, but specificity for interstitial nephritis is only about 80%. Other causes of AKI in which eosinophiluria is relatively common are rapidly progressive glomerulonephritis and renal atheroemboli. Discontinuation of the potential causative agent is a mainstay of therapy.

Abdominal Compartment Syndrome

Abdominal compartment syndrome is a clinical diagnosis in the setting of increased intra-abdominal pressure—pressures below 10 mm Hg generally rule it out, while pressures above 25 mm Hg make it likely. Baseline blood pressure and abdominal wall compliance influence the amount of intra-abdominal pressure that can be tolerated. Surgical decompression is the only definitive therapy and should be undertaken before irreversible end-organ damage occurs.

Renal Replacement Therapy

Continuous renal replacement therapy forms the mainstay of replacement therapy in critically ill patients who often cannot tolerate standard hemodialysis due to hemodynamic instability. Standard intermittent hemodialysis is not generally appropriate for hypotensive patients, but some centers modify standard dialysis (primarily by prolonging it for many hours) and this may be a reasonable alternative in settings where continuous renal replacement therapy cannot be accomplished. Peritoneal dialysis is not usually sufficient. Mortality in the setting of acute renal failure in the critically ill is high (50%–60%). Renal recovery in survivors may be as high as 90%, but recent studies suggest that sustained renal failure or incomplete renal recovery is more common than previously thought (as many as 50% of survivors do not return to baseline renal function following an episode of acute renal failure).

Pearls of Care

1. Acute kidney injury (AKI) is common in patients presenting to emergency departments; monitor serum creatinine and urine output in all patients at risk.
2. Use modified RIFLE (AKIN) criteria to diagnose and stage AKI.
3. Discontinue all unnecessary nephrotoxic agents in high-risk patients and in those with AKI as nephrotoxins will impair recovery.
4. Ensure adequate circulating blood volume as in all critically ill patients but avoid volume overload in patients with AKI.
5. Consider early RRT for patients with RIFLE-I (injury) or greater AKI. Start therapy before complications of AKI occur.

Selected Readings

Bellomo R, Ronco C, Kellum JA, Mehta RL, Palevsky P. Acute renal failure—definition, outcome measures, animal models, fluid therapy and information technology needs: the Second International Consensus Conference of the Acute Dialysis Quality Initiative (ADQI) Group. *Crit Care* 2004;8:R204–R212.

Kellum JA. Acute kidney injury. *Crit Care Med* 2008;36:S141–S145.

Uchino S, Kellum JA, Bellomo R, et al. Acute renal failure in critically ill patients: a multinational, multicenter study. *JAMA* 2005;294:813–818.

Chapter 7

Coma and Altered Mental Status

J. Stephen Huff and Robert D. Stevens

Introduction

Coma reflects brain failure, either from a primary process within the central nervous system (CNS) or from interaction of the CNS with systemic metabolic processes. Coma is a sign that CNS uncoupling, dysfunction, or destruction has occurred. The process leading to the altered mental status may be either static or dynamic, but often the time course is unknown. The physician must rapidly detect and either ameliorate or correct ongoing destructive processes. The clinician must simultaneously engage in resuscitative and diagnostic interventions. Brief assessment of responsiveness and stabilization are the initial steps.

Coma is usually a transient state. Patients with coma from brain injury or illness will die, recover awareness, or evolve into a state of impaired consciousness such as the minimally conscious or vegetative state.[1] Altered mental status may be a prodrome of coma. Accurate diagnosis is needed to ensure appropriate treatment and prognosis.

Definition of Terms

To the emergency physician, assessment of the patient with altered mental status requires some knowledge of the baseline level of functioning of the patient. Deviations in mental functioning from the baseline state span a clinical spectrum, ranging from mild confusion, delirium, stupor, to coma. As the most severe derangement in consciousness, coma may be defined operationally as an eyes-closed unresponsive state. Both arousal (wakefulness) and awareness (content of consciousness) are severely impaired. Within coma, a spectrum of behaviors may include limb movements (localizing or withdrawal), reflexive movements, and nonpurposeful movements (extension or flexion). The Glasgow Coma Scale (Table 7.1) is a common tool to quantify depth of coma.

Conceptually, coma results from brainstem dysfunction with disruption of arousal functions, or global dysfunction of cerebral and higher cortical functions.

Table 7.1 Glasgow Coma Scale

Eye opening	
Spontaneous	4
To speech	3
To pain	2
None	1
Best motor response	
Obeys	6
Localizes	5
Withdraws	4
Abnormal flexion	3
Extensor response	2
None	1
Best verbal response	
Oriented	5
Confused conversation	4
Inappropriate words	3
Incomprehensible words	2
None	1

The two processes often coexist. Unilateral cerebral impairment results in focal neurological abnormalities (stroke syndromes) and not coma.

Acute coma may persist, or it may resolve into wakefulness. Intermediate outcomes include the vegetative state or the minimally conscious state.[1,2] The vegetative state is characterized by wakefulness without awareness. The brainstem systems responsible for alertness continue to function, but cortical and thalamic systems are structurally or functionally impaired. For example, eyes may be open, but the patient does not respond to surroundings. The minimally conscious state is characterized by unresponsiveness punctuated by intermittent evidence for awareness. The patient may intermittently but inconsistently follow simple commands, gesture "yes" or "no" answers, visually pursue objects, or show other signs of responsiveness.[1]

Clinical Syndromes and Pathophysiology

Full consciousness—awareness and alertness—requires functioning neuronal systems residing in the cerebral cortex and brainstem. Dysfunction of the brainstem, dysfunction of both cerebral hemispheres, or global CNS dysfunction (both hemispheres and brainstem) may result in coma or altered mental status. Dysfunction of one cerebral hemisphere (for example, stroke in internal carotid or middle cerebral artery distribution) may alter the content of consciousness, but it should not cause coma. Stroke could lead to coma if additional processes are active, such as cerebral edema with brainstem compression.

The brain is metabolically demanding, requiring constant provision of oxygen and glucose as metabolic substrates. Low levels or impaired delivery of oxygen or glucose will cause immediate impairment of global CNS function. Additionally, many other processes may interfere with the complex neurochemical and neuroelectrical function of the CNS. Toxins, either exogenous or endogenous as with metabolic encephalopathies, may alter consciousness due to interference with neurotransmission or other mechanisms.

Maintenance of regional and global cerebral blood flow depends on cerebral perfusion pressure (CPP) and also can be affected by acidosis, hypercapnia, and hypocapnia. CPP is approximated by the equation CPP = MAP − ICP, where MAP is the mean arterial pressure and ICP is the intracranial pressure. Although cerebral blood flow is maintained over a range of CPP (50–150 mm Hg in healthy adults), even transient low blood pressure or shock states can result in brain ischemia. Increased ICP also will reduce CPP. Strategies to lower ICP must preserve MAP in order to improve CPP. MAP is best measured by arterial catheter but can be approximated by [systolic BP + (2 × diastolic BP)]/3. ICP measurement cannot be estimated accurately without invasive ICP monitor placement. Papilledema or retinal hemorrhages suggest increased ICP, but increased ICP may occur without recognizable ocular signs.

Localized or compartmental increases in ICP may result in herniation syndromes. The most recognizable of these is uncal or temporal lobe herniation syndrome, with medial shift of the temporal lobe. This results in physical or functional impairment of cranial nerve III, usually on the side of the expanding or shifting medial temporal lobe. The full syndrome consists of ipsilateral mydriasis, impaired extraocular movements (with Cr N III impairment, unopposed Cr N VI activity, and resulting depression and abduction of the eye), a reduced level of consciousness, and contralateral hemiparesis and upper motor neuron signs (due to ipsilateral cerebral peduncle compression). The observation that use of osmolar agents or surgical decompression at times resolves herniation syndromes implies that the impairment may be physiological rather than structural.[3,4]

General Management

Systematic investigation of the cause of altered mental status or coma (Table 7.2) should proceed concurrently with treatment of immediately life-threatening conditions (Table 7.3).

Although the etiology of altered mental status or coma is often discernible from history, the patient usually cannot provide that history. Providers should seek collateral history from emergency medical service providers, caregivers, family, eyewitnesses, and any other potential sources. Medical records may

Table 7.2 Etiologies of Coma

Coma from causes affecting the brain diffusely

Encephalopathies
  Hypoxic
  Hypercarbia/respiratory failure
  Metabolic
  Hepatic
  Electrolyte disturbances
  Uremic
  Hypertensive
  Endocrine

Toxins

Environmental

Deficiency states

Sepsis

Coma from primary CNS disease or trauma

CNS trauma
  Vascular disease
  Anterior circulation ischemic stroke with brainstem compression
  Posterior circulation ischemic stroke
  Intracranial hemorrhages
    ICH
    Cerebellar hemorrhage

CNS infections
  Encephalitis
  Meningitis

Neoplasms with hemorrhage or mass effect

Seizures
Generalized convulsive status epilepticus
Nonconvulsive status epilepticus

CNS, central nervous system; ICH, intracranial hemorrhage.

provide clues of existing medical problems or reveal recently prescribed medications. A history of seizure disorder or seizures witnessed before the unresponsiveness might suggest transformed or subtle generalized status epilepticus. Occupational history or the whereabouts of the patient at time of symptom onset may provide clues to occupational or environmental exposures. The tempo of onset may be helpful; abrupt onset of coma or altered consciousness may suggest seizures, cerebrovascular, or cardiac etiologies. Metabolic encephalopathies may have a more gradual onset of symptoms over minutes or hours.

Physical exam should first assess airway, breathing, and circulation. Some obvious physical findings such as cyanosis or apnea will dictate immediate interventions. However, clinical judgment about depth of respirations, ability to guard

Table 7.3 Initial Evaluation of Coma

History
    Collateral sources (family, emergency medical service, witnesses)
    Medical record

ABC's
    Immediate supportive care to reverse hypotension or hypoxemia
    Detect and treat hypoglycemia (most common cause of coma in the emergency department)

Establish level of consciousness
    Glasgow Coma Scale
    Detailed response to verbal, tactile, or noxious stimuli

Consider structural etiologies
    External signs of trauma
    Cranial nerve abnormalities
    CT scan
    Other imaging as indicated (CT angiography, CT-perfusion, MRI)

Consider nonstructural etiologies
    History of gradual onset
    Vital sign abnormalities suggesting systemic disease
    Metabolic derangements (laboratory profile)
    Infectious etiologies (lumbar puncture as indicated)
    Nonconvulsive status epilepticus (EEG)
    Toxicological profile

Specific treatments
    Glucose (with thiamine in setting of nutritional deficiencies)
    Hypertension management (stroke, subarachnoid hemorrhage, ICH)
    Naloxone
    Antibiotics (with dexamethasone if meningitis)

Specific management for increased ICP
    Mannitol or other osmotic therapy
    Avoid prolonged hyperventilation
    Steroids for neoplasm-associated edema
    Surgical management

CT, computed tomography; EEG, electroencephalogram; ICH, intracranial hemorrhage; ICP, intracranial pressure; MRI, magnetic resonance imaging.

the airway, and stability of other vital signs will guide immediate actions. Airway management is covered in Chapter 15. Hypotension and shock are covered in Chapter 16.

Next, establish level of consciousness. A patient with eyes closed who remains unresponsive to stimulation and without appropriate movements or facial expressions is comatose. Use graded stimuli to confirm the unresponsiveness. Assess reactions to verbal, tactile, and then noxious stimuli. Noxious stimuli that are intense but do not cause tissue injury include sternal rub, nail bed pressure, and pressure on the supraorbital ridges or other bony prominences. There are no data to recommend one maneuver one over another.

The Glasgow Coma Scale is a brief assessment tool to quantify best motor response, best eye-opening response, and best verbal response (Table 7.1). A variety of abnormal reflex postures, including flexor and extensor responses, may be present and a description of the best motor response should be noted. Distinguishing between purposeful and nonpurposeful activity may be difficult at times. Generally, movements across the midline may be thought to be purposeful or semipurposeful, while reflex movements do not cross the patient's midline. For example, reaching toward an endotracheal tube may be purposeful, while simple flexion of the upper extremity is likely reflexive. Abnormal movements might reflect seizure activity or abnormal reflex posturing. At times, seizure activity may be subtle with only facial or eye movements, or at times with absence of any motor activity even when epileptiform activity is observable electrographically.

Bedside glucose testing should be performed in all patients with intervention as needed. Though a universally accepted definition of hypoglycemia is lacking, it would seem prudent to administer dextrose (25 mL of dextrose 50%) in patients with bedside test results of less than 70 mg/dL. Thiamine 100 mg should be administered to patients with potential risk of nutritional deficiencies such as alcoholism, poor nutritional status, malabsorption states, or a history of bariatric surgery. If elements of the opiate toxidrome are present (bradypnea, miotic pupils), naloxone should be administered at 0.4 mg to 0.8 mg intravenously to be repeated as needed.

Survey the head, neck, chest, and extremities for unusual rashes or traumatic injuries. The cervical spine should be immobilized if there is suspicion for trauma with subsequent imaging of spine and brain.

Assess cranial nerves in order to gauge brainstem functions. The gag response has likely been assessed during airway evaluation. Pupillary size, reactivity, and symmetry should be assessed. The corneal reflex is either present or absent. Like the pupillary response, this has both direct and consensual components. A hand clap or other loud noise may provoke a reflex blink. Though not often performed in the emergency department, assessment of oculocephalic or oculovestibular reflexes provides information regarding the brainstem, frontal eye fields, and interconnections. Cranial nerve function survey tests the integrity of the afferent cranial nerve, brainstem nuclei, interneuronal pathways, efferent cranial nerve, and supratentorial modulation.

Persistent deviation of the eyes may indicate seizure activity, postictal phenomena, or impaired extraocular movements from central damage to cranial nerves, brainstem, or cerebral structures. An old axiom is that eyes deviate toward the side of a destructive cerebral lesion (e.g. stroke) and away from an excitatory lesion (e.g. seizure).

Hypothermia is rarely the cause of unresponsiveness, but mild hypothermia is common in sepsis and other metabolic encephalopathies. Though central fevers do exist, these are rare at presentation and remain a diagnosis of exclusion.

Elevated body temperature suggests possible infection or may be part of a toxidrome. In the appropriate environment heat stress is another possibility. Status epilepticus may cause elevated body temperature from excessive motor activity.

Tachycardias may reflect sepsis, toxidromes, hypovolemia, or a primary cardiac problem. Bradycardia may be caused by a primary cardiac problem or hypoxia. Bradycardia with hypertension may indicate elevated intracranial pressure (ICP). Rapid deep respirations may reflect compensation for metabolic acidosis or central hyperventilation.

Response to initial stabilization and resuscitative maneuvers will guide further evaluation. For example, a patient with hypoglycemia (still the most common cause of coma in US emergency departments) who fully awakens with dextrose administration and gives a history of diabetes and dietary irregularity may require no further evaluation. For the patient with persistent unresponsiveness, initial laboratory testing should be obtained, including electrolytes, liver function tests, hematologic panel, arterial blood gas, and initial toxicologic measurements including blood-alcohol level. Urinalysis and cultures of the blood and urine may be obtained.

The differential diagnosis of coma is vast (Table 7.2), but initial evaluation often assigns patients into three preliminary categories of coma: (1) likely structural, (2) likely nonstructural, or (3) etiology unclear. Structural coma is suggested by asymmetric findings on physical examination. For example, unilateral pupillary dilation or asymmetric extraocular movements may suggest posterior communicating artery aneurysm rupture or uncal herniation as described earlier. A nonstructural cause of coma is suggested by progressive onset of symptoms or perhaps from a history of medication use, alcohol ingestion, or an environmental toxic exposure. Neurological impairment is global and findings on physical examination tend to be symmetric. However, the absence of physical examination responses does not always allow distinction between structural and metabolic coma. For example, a metabolic or infectious cause of coma may evolve into a structural problem with onset of cerebral edema. Further diagnostic strategies and management proceed from the likely differential diagnosis.

Unless a readily reversible cause of coma is discovered with rapid improvement in the patient's clinical status, cranial computed tomography (CT) scanning should be obtained to exclude structural lesions. Noncontrast CT scan remains a sensitive screening test for intracranial hemorrhage (ICH), subarachnoid hemorrhage, edema, and mass effect. Perhaps the most significant limitation of noncontrast cranial CT is the insensitivity to acute ischemia. Some hours may be required for development of even early signs of ischemia such as sulcal effacement and other signs of edema. CT angiography (with or without CT perfusion), or diffusion- and perfusion-weighted magnetic resonance imaging (MRI) may be useful in this setting. There are no data to guide the clinician in specific cases, and recommendations at different institutions will likely vary.

Herniation syndromes may also be apparent on CT scan and may include significant shift of midline structures. Frequently there is a correlation between an abnormal neurological examination and radiographic abnormalities; but exceptions occur in which patients have normal neurological examination despite significant brain shift or brain herniation on CT.[5]

Suspected increased ICP is treated by elevating the head and keeping the head in the midline. Steroids have no effect on ICP in head injury or stroke but may be effective in edema associated with neoplasms or brain abscesses. If increased ICP is detected, any hyperventilation should be transient and mild with reduction of $PaCO_2$ to only 30–35 mm Hg to avoid cerebral ischemia. Osmotic agents include mannitol and hypertonic saline; mannitol is commonly used in dosages of 0.5–1 g/kg bolus.

Controversies in Management

The timing of lumbar puncture to detect central nervous system infections is often deferred pending radiology studies. If high pretest probability of central nervous system infection exists, antibiotic therapy should be initiated to cover likely pathogens based on empiric age-guided recommendations. Modify antibiotic selection based on recent hospitalizations and other risk factors for antibiotic-resistant organisms. If acute bacterial meningitis is likely, consider adjunctive treatment with dexamethasone (10 mg in adults) when antibiotic therapy is initiated.

Treatment of hypertension in the comatose patient is controversial. Excessive or rapid lowering of blood pressure may diminish CPP and worsen focal or regional brain ischemia particularly when there is a history of hypertension. In ischemic stroke, titratable anti-hypertensive agents should be initiated for blood pressure greater than 185/110 mm Hg if thrombolytic therapy is a consideration, and greater than 220/120 mm Hg in subjects who are not candidates for thrombolysis. Patients with a subarchnoid hemorrhage and an unsecured aneurysm should have high blood pressure treated. While there are no rigorous evidence-based guidelines and local practices vary, a systolic blood pressure <140 mm Hg is a common target. In the patient with ICH, definitive data are lacking, but current guidelines recommend targeting a blood pressure <180/130 mm Hg in the absence of intracranial hypertension.[6]

Routine electroencephalography (EEG) is rare in the emergency department, but recent studies have advocated for routine EEG for comatose patients in the intensive care unit. Epileptiform activity has unexpectedly been identified in many comatose patients. Whether this is the cause or an effect of the underlying condition is not clear, but untreated generalized status epilepticus may worsen neuronal injury. Consider EEG for patients receiving pharmacologic paralysis as part of management and for patients with observed seizures who fail to show improvement in consciousness after approximately 30 minutes.

Management of serum glucose in patients with neurological injury remains controversial. Certainly persistent hyperglycemia has been associated with worse outcomes in patients with stroke. However, aggressive management of moderate hyperglycemia increases the likelihood of hypoglycemic episodes and should be avoided. Treatment of hyperglycemia >200 mg/dL is reasonable in most situations.

Prolonged use of narcotic antagonists may be difficult to titrate and should not be a substitute for airway management. Requirement for repeated naloxone administration may indicate the presence of a long-acting opiate such as methadone. Naloxone infusions have been used but have fallen from favor because of the chance of precipitating narcotic withdrawal. With mixed ingestions including acetaminophen, use of N–acetylcysteine is recommended. Consultation with a clinical toxicologist is advised.

Prognostication of ultimate neurologic function in patients after cardiac arrest is impossible in the emergency department and no definitive prognostication may be attempted for 48–72 hours post arrest. Consideration of postcardiac arrest care is discussed in Chapter 8.

Brain death determination in the emergency department is controversial because a period of observation and reassessment is a critical part of brain death assessment.

Pearls of Care

1. Supportive care and stabilization with attention to the ABC's is vital.
2. Initial clinical evaluation allows many patients to be assigned with a likely cause of coma, but there should be a low threshold to obtain neuroimaging to exclude structural etiologies should diagnostic doubts remain.
3. Nonconvulsive status epilepticus requires EEG monitoring to detect. Suspect this in patients who fail to become alert within 20 to 30 minutes following cessation of seizure activity.
4. Prognosis after resuscitation from cardiac arrest is not possible in the time frame of patient care in the emergency department.
5. Advanced neuroimaging such as CT-angiography, CT-perfusion, and MRI studies may be required in selected cases of patients in coma.

References

1. Bernat JL. Current controversies in states of chronic unconsciousness. *Neurol Clin Prac* 2010;75(Suppl 1):S33–S38.

2. Rosenberg RN. Consciousness, coma, and brain death—2009. *JAMA* 2009;301(11):1172–1174.

3. Maramattom BV, Wijdicks EFM. Uncal herniation. *Arch Neurol* 2005;62(12):1932–1950.

4. Koenig MA, Bryan M, Lewin JL, et al. Reversal of transtentorial herniation with hypertonic saline. *Neurology* 2008;70(13):1023–1029.

5. Probst MA, Baraff LJ, Hoffman JR, et al. Can patients with brain herniation on cranial computed tomography have a normal neurologic exam? *Acad Emerg Med* 2009;16(2):145–150.

6. Morganstern LB, Hemphill JC, 3rd, Anderson C, et al. Guidelines for the management of spontaneous intracerebral hemorrhage: a guideline for healthcare professionals fropm the American Heart Association/American Stroke Association. *Stroke* 2010;41(9):2108–2129.

Selected Readings

Brown EN, Lydic R, Schiff ND. Mechanisms of disease: general anesthesia, sleep, and coma. *N Engl J Med* 2010;363(27):2638–2650.

Emergency Neurological Life Support (ENLS) management algorithms. Available at: http://www.neurocriticalcare.org

Wijdicks EF, Varelas PN, Gronseth GS, et al. Evidence-based guideline update: determining brain death in adults. *Neurology* 2010;74(23):1911–1918.

Young BG. Neurologic prognosis after cardiac arrest. *N Engl J Med* 2009;361(6):605–611.

Chapter 8

Post–Cardiac Arrest Care

Stephen Trzeciak

Introduction

Sudden cardiac arrest is the most common fatal manifestation of cardiovascular disease, and it represents one of the leading causes of death worldwide. Even if effective circulation is restored with emergency interventions such as cardio-pulmonary resuscitation (CPR) and defibrillation, more than half of resuscitated patients do not survive to hospital discharge, and many who survive sustain crip-pling neurological sequelae. Anoxic brain injury is the primary factor contributing to death and disability in postresuscitation patients. It is now clear that interven-tions initiated *after* the return of pulses can improve outcomes. Specifically, the discovery that therapeutic hypothermia (TH) can improve neurological function in postresuscitation patients has dramatically transformed the classical thinking about post–cardiac arrest brain injury. We now recognize that this potentially devastating condition is in fact treatable. Given a tremendous opportunity for a meaningful impact on outcome for critically ill postresuscitation patients, it is essential for emergency physicians to have a sound understanding of the basic principles of post–cardiac arrest care.

Definition of Terms

Cardiac arrest: the cessation of effective cardiac mechanical activity as confirmed by the absence of signs of circulation.

Cardiopulmonary resuscitation (CPR): an emergency procedure involving a combination of chest compressions and rescue breathing delivered to victims thought to be in cardiac arrest with the goal of achieving return of spontane-ous circulation.

Post–cardiac arrest syndrome: the state of critical illness following return of spontaneous circulation from cardiac arrest that is characterized by whole-body ischemia-reperfusion injury, and typically manifests with post–cardiac arrest brain injury, a systemic proinflammatory response, reversible myocardial depression, and possibly acute coronary syndrome.

Reperfusion injury: tissue and organ system injury that occurs when circulation is restored to tissues after a period of ischemia. Reperfusion injury is character-ized by inflammatory changes and oxidative stress.

Return of spontaneous circulation (ROSC): restoration of sustained perfusing cardiac activity (i.e., restoration of a palpable pulse) after cardiac arrest.

Therapeutic hypothermia: a treatment strategy that reduces a patient's body temperature (typically to 33°C–34°C) in order to help reduce the risk of permanent brain injury after resuscitation from cardiac arrest.

Clinical Syndrome

Resuscitation from cardiac arrest involves whole-body ischemia-reperfusion injury with the following main clinical manifestations: (1) post–cardiac arrest brain injury, (2) profound systemic inflammation, (3) reversible myocardial depression, and often (4) acute coronary syndrome. This clinical syndrome was originally termed by Negovsky in the 1970s as "postresuscitation disease," but the more commonly used term today is *post–cardiac arrest syndrome*.

Post–Cardiac Arrest Brain Injury

One of the most important principles of post–cardiac arrest care is the concept that cellular injury after reperfusion is a dynamic process. The initial ischemic event has already occurred and can no longer be mitigated, but the severity of the reperfusion injury is potentially modifiable. Neuronal cell death in laboratory investigations develops over 48–72 hours after ROSC. These hours are a window of opportunity in which the brain injury from cardiac arrest can be treated.

The brain is particularly susceptible to ischemia/reperfusion injury. The pathophysiological mechanisms occurring in the brain with reperfusion include mitochondrial dysfunction and disruption of cerebral energy metabolism, loss of cellular calcium ion homeostasis, neuronal excitotoxicity, triggering of apoptosis, and possibly cerebral microcirculatory dysfunction. These processes cause injury to neurons over hours and perhaps days and are potential therapeutic targets. Initiating therapy in the emergency department (ED) increases the time available to modify the natural history of this syndrome. Patients who exhibit signs of poor neurological function at the time of ROSC do have potential for meaningful recovery. After the implementation of therapeutic hypothermia, up to 20%–50% of comatose patients with post–cardiac arrest syndrome at the time of reperfusion have a favorable outcome. Resolution of coma occurs over days after ROSC, and neurological recovery may last for months.

Systemic Inflammatory Response

Whole-body ischemia/reperfusion is a potent trigger of systemic inflammation. ROSC triggers sharp increases in circulating cytokines and other markers of the inflammatory response. Accordingly, the post–cardiac arrest syndrome has been called a "sepsis-like" state. The clinical manifestations of profound systemic inflammation may include marked hemodynamic effects such as arterial hypotension similar to septic shock. Hemodynamic instability is present in approximately 50% of patients admitted to an intensive care unit after cardiac arrest, and thus the need for hemodynamic support (e.g., vasoactive agents, advanced hemodynamic monitoring) should be anticipated. While the systemic inflammatory response can certainly induce or exacerbate arterial hypotension, an equally important contributor to hemodynamic instability after ROSC is myocardial stunning.

Reversible Myocardial Dysfunction

Severe, but reversible, myocardial dysfunction is commonly observed after ROSC from cardiac arrest. The etiology of this global myocardial stunning is thought to be ischemia/reperfusion injury, perhaps exacerbated by electrical injury from defibrillation, if applied. While the myocardial dysfunction can be expected to occur in the absence of coronary insufficiency or infarct, myocardial ischemia from an acute coronary syndrome also should be considered as a potential cause of myocardial depression. Myocardial stunning may last for 24–48 hours and may be responsive to support with inotropic agents.

Acute Coronary Syndrome

The most common etiology of sudden cardiac arrest is acute coronary syndrome. Therefore, it is imperative for clinicians to have a high clinical suspicion of acute myocardial ischemia as the inciting event for the cardiac arrest when no other etiology is clearly apparent. While the presence of ST-segment myocardial infarction is an obvious indication for emergent revascularization, other more subtle abnormalities may be found on the electrocardiogram and indicate the presence of an ischemic event, either with or without infarct, as the cause of the arrest. Early cardiac catheterization and reperfusion therapy should be considered (see next section).

General Management

The current American Heart Association recommendations for optimal immediate post–cardiac arrest care (Fig. 8.1) are based on four essential elements:

• Therapeutic hypothermia to reduce the risk of permanent brain injury
• Critical care support to optimize hemodynamic status and vital organ perfusion
• Interventional cardiac catheterization capability for possible percutaneous coronary intervention (if necessary)
• An evidence-based approach to neurological prognostication to prevent inappropriately early judgements of poor neurological prognosis

Therapeutic Hypothermia

Therapeutic hypothermia involves a strategy to reduce the body temperature of a cardiac arrest victim after a pulse is restored for the purpose of improving post–cardiac arrest brain injury. The goal for body temperature is typically

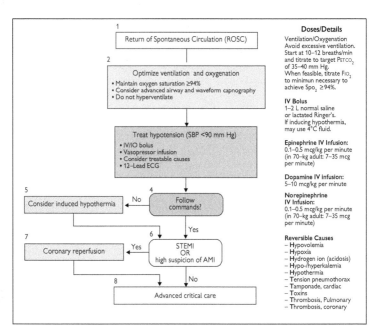

Figure 8.1 The American Heart Association treatment algorithm for post–cardiac arrest care. AMI, acute myocardial infarction; ECG, electrocardiogram; IO, intraosseous; IV, intravenous; ROSC, return of spontaneous circulation; SBP, systolic blood pressure; STEMI, ST-segment elevation myocardial infarction.

32°C–34°C for 12–24 hours after ROSC. The mechanisms by which TH may confer protection from reperfusion injury to the brain include the following: reduction in cerebral metabolism and mitochondrial dysfunction, improvement of bioenergetic homeostasis, reduction of apoptosis, reduction in oxygen free radical production, reduced neuronal excitotoxicity, improved calcium ion hemostasis, and potentially seizure suppression. Two landmark clinical trials of therapeutic hypothermia after ROSC showed improved neurological outcome for patients treated with therapeutic hypothermia (compared to normothermia) among patients with out-of-hospital cardiac arrest who had ventricular fibrillation (VF) as the initial rhythm. The American Heart Association recommends TH for adult patients who are comatose after ROSC following out-of-hospital VF cardiac arrest, targeting a temperature of 32°C–34°C for 12–24 hours (Class 1 recommendation). For patients with other initial rhythms or in-hospital cardiac arrest, TH may also be considered (Class 2B recommendation).

Appropriate patient selection for TH is imperative. If a patient lacks a meaningful response to verbal commands after ROSC is achieved, this indicates that the patient has demonstrated brain injury and TH should be strongly considered. If a patient is clearly following commands immediately after ROSC (which can occur after relatively short no-flow times with effective CPR), then significant brain injury is less likely and TH may be reasonably withheld.

There are three phases of TH: induction, maintenance, and rewarming. In the ED setting, only the induction phase of therapy is typically of concern. Therapeutic hypothermia should be initiated as soon as possible after ROSC using any of the various methods for hypothermia induction. These include external cooling devices, intravascular cooling catheters, or a combination of both. External cooling methods include ice packs and cooling blankets. Cold (4°C) intravenous saline infusion can supplement both intravascular and external devices for induction. Devices specifically intended for targeted temperature management have computer modules that regulate the flow of cold fluid through the devices and are based on a feedback loop with the body temperature of the patient. One of the advantages of these types of devices is limiting the risk of "overshoot" (temperature ≤31°C). Overshoot may occur more commonly with ice packs and conventional cooling blankets than with the cooling devices. A disadvantage of the automated devices compared to methods that do not use advanced technology is cost.

Shivering is very common and can be detrimental to the patient by making goal temperature more difficult, or impossible, to achieve. Therefore, immediate recognition and treatment of shivering is imperative. Adequate sedation and analgesics are essential components of TH, especially the induction phase. Often the administration of additional sedative and/or opioid agents will be sufficient to ameliorate shivering. If shivering persists, neuromuscular blocking agents may be required. If neuromuscular blocking agents are used, they are often only necessary in the induction phase of TH when the temperature is dropping at a rapid rate. Once target temperature is achieved, patients often stop shivering. Therefore, it is prudent to try to limit neuromuscular blocking agents to the induction phase of therapeutic hypothermia, as they likely can be withheld thereafter. Unnecessarily prolonged neuromuscular blockade should be avoided, because prolonged neuromuscular weakness may persist after discontinuation. This could potentially cloud the patient's neurological assessment at a later time point. When using neuromuscular blocking agents for the induction of TH, their administration may be titrated to the resolution of shivering rather than complete paralysis, which may result in a much lower dose of neuromuscular blocker being administered. Duration of neuromuscular blockade can be prolonged significantly during TH due to decreased drug metabolism.

If TH is not initiated for any reason, fever is clearly detrimental (presumably by increasing cerebral metabolic rate) and must be avoided. Fever is not uncommon in the post–cardiac arrest population because of the intense proinflammatory response to ischemia/reperfusion and must be treated aggressively with conventional antipyretic therapies and techniques.

Physicians need to be aware of potential complications that can be associated with TH. These include coagulopathy, hyperglycemia, bradycardia, increased risk of secondary infection, electrolyte shifts, and hypovolemia related to a "cold diuresis." Fortunately, when these complications do occur, they are usually not severe. In risk-benefit decisions regarding whether to use TH for a patient with post–cardiac arrest syndrome, the risk of complications related to TH is typically greatly outweighed by the increased risk of permanent brain injury if TH is withheld. Ongoing, noncompressible bleeding is perhaps the strongest contraindication to TH.

Critical Care Support

The American Heart Association guidelines recommend optimization of cardiopulmonary function and vital organ perfusion after ROSC to reduce the risk of multiorgan injury (Table 8.1). Hemodynamic instability is common (~50% of patients) after resuscitation from cardiac arrest, and is associated with sharply higher mortality among post–cardiac arrest patients. To date, there have been no clinical trials of hemodynamic optimization strategies targeting specific goals or hemodynamic indices after ROSC. Despite the absence of experimental data on this topic, it is prudent to be aggressive about raising the blood pressure in patients who remain markedly hypotensive after resuscitation. The optimal blood pressure goal after ROSC is currently unclear. An echocardiogram may be helpful in hemodynamic assessment in the early post–cardiac arrest period to determine whether global myocardial depression is present. If present, the patient may benefit from support with an inotropic agent or mechanical augmentation (e.g., intra-aortic balloon counterpulsation) until the myocardial function recovers. However, when needed, clinicians should use agents with beta-adrenergic properties cautiously because of the arrhythmogenic potential. In summary, current expert opinion advocates a general approach in which clinical acumen is used to optimize the patient's hemodynamic status and global organ perfusion. Specific optimal goals of therapy or optimal hemodynamic targets have yet to be elucidated.

Hyperventilation should be avoided because of the potential for cerebral vasoconstriction with hypocarbia and associated risk of ongoing cerebral ischemia. In addition, hyperventilation could have major hemodynamic effects in this population. Overly aggressive ventilation (e.g., "overbagging" the patient prior to initiation of mechanical ventilation or excessively high minute ventilation set on the ventilator) can cause intrinsic positive end-expiratory pressure (PEEP), which can increase intrathoracic pressure and reduce cardiac output.

Exposure to hyperoxemia (excessively high arterial partial pressure of oxygen) has been associated with poor clinical outcome in observational studies of adult patients resuscitated from cardiac arrest. The scientific rationale for potential harmful effects of hyperoxemia is supported by numerous laboratory studies showing that post-ROSC hyperoxemia worsens histopathological changes in the brain as well as functional neurological deficits among animals resuscitated from cardiac arrest. Therefore, there may be a paradox with regard to reoxygenation of the injured brain, where persistent hypoxemia could exacerbate anoxic brain injury, but excessive oxygen delivery could worsen reperfusion injury, presumably by an acceleration of oxygen free radical formation. No

Table 8.1 Critical Interventions after Cardiac Arrest

Cardiovascular
  Assess for STEMI or acute coronary syndrome
  Reperfusion therapy/PCI if indicated
  Support blood pressure with volume, pressors, or inotropes

Pulmonary
  Reduce FiO_2 as tolerated
  Avoid hyperventilation

Neurological
  Assess coma
  Initiate hypothermia if indicated
  Shivering suppression
  Monitor for seizures

Metabolic
  Metabolic acidosis will correct with restoration of perfusion
  Correct electrolyte disturbances

PCI, percutaneous coronary intervention; STEMI, ST-segment myocardial infarction.

clinical trials of a strategy employing rapid downward titration of supplemental oxygen ("controlled reoxygenation") have been performed to date, but current expert opinion advocates limiting exposure to unnecessarily high levels of supplemental oxygen and maintaining arterial oxygen saturation in the 94%–96% range, if possible.

Seizures are not uncommon after anoxic brain injury, and it is important to be vigilant in clinical assessment for any motor responses that could represent seizure activity so that it can be treated promptly. Continuous electroencephalography monitoring (if available) can be useful, especially if continuous administration of neuromuscular blocking agents becomes necessary for any reason.

Coronary Interventions

Patients with evidence of an ST-segment myocardial infarction (STEMI) on electrocardiogram should receive emergent cardiac catheterization and revascularization. However, as many as 50% of patients without STEMI but a strong clinical suspicion for a coronary event may have a coronary lesion on angiography that warrants intervention. In patients with no obvious noncardiac etiology of cardiac arrest, a clinical suspicion of coronary ischemia, and an abnormal electrocardiogram after ROSC, urgent consultation with an interventional cardiologist is warranted. Immediate cardiac catheterization and coronary angiography should be strongly considered in any post–cardiac arrest patient in which acute coronary syndrome is strongly suspected as the inciting event. Recent studies have demonstrated the feasibility of inducing hypothermia simultaneously with emergent percutaneous coronary intervention.

Neurological Prognostication

Although neurological prognostication is not typically performed in the emergency department setting, it is important for the emergency physician to have a general understanding of the approach to prognostication so that a cohesive plan of care can be formulated and communicated both to the family and to the subsequent care providers in the intensive care unit. Neurological prognostication is notoriously challenging for the first few days after ROSC. Although many neurological signs may suggest a poor prognosis, very few are reliable enough upon which to base neurological prognostication until 72 hours or more after ROSC. In general, a prudent approach to neurological prognostication after cardiac arrest is to avoid making inappropriately early projections of futility that could dissuade aggressive management, but at the same time avoid generating expectations for recovery among caregivers or family that could be unrealistic.

Key Controversies

Is Therapeutic Hypothermia Beneficial in Patients with Non–Ventricular Fibrillation Initial Rhythms?

The landmark clinical trials of TH only included patients with VF cardiac arrest. Whether or not TH is beneficial in patients with non-VF initial rhythms (e.g., pulseless electrical activity, asystole) remains controversial. Some of the available observational data have suggested that application of TH is not associated with improved outcome in this population. There is no biologic rationale for post–cardiac arrest brain injury to respond differently to TH based on the initial rhythm. Rather, this overall poor prognosis for patients with non-VF initial rhythm (likely related to the underlying etiology of arrest) creates difficulty in showing statistical differences among groups. Given that (1) no other therapeutic options exist for post–cardiac arrest brain injury, (2) complications associated with TH are usually not severe relative to the overall clinical picture, and (3) no clinical data report lower survival associated with TH, TH should be considered when a patient with non-VF initial rhythm is not following commands after ROSC. For this population, TH is a Class 2B recommendation in guidelines from the American Heart Association.

How Fast Must Therapeutic Hypothermia Be Initiated in Order to Be Beneficial?

Some observational data in human subjects resuscitated from cardiac arrest and one randomized trial of paramedic cooling in the field versus waiting until ED arrival for TH induction have reported no significant association between faster TH and improved outcome. However, these clinical reports should be interpreted with some caution. In the randomized trial, both groups had identical mean body temperatures after 1 hour, suggesting that the earlier attempts at TH induction in the field may have been insufficient. In observational studies, the association between time to target temperature and outcome can potentially be confounded by the patient's baseline body temperature after ROSC. For example, moribund patients with exceptionally poor prognosis are often spontaneously hypothermic after ROSC and thus can be expected to have a shorter time to target temperature. Taken together, there is insufficient clinical data at the present time in order to make an evidence-based judgment on this question. Laboratory investigations indicate that the benefits of TH decline after delays of 4–6 hours. Although the optimal therapeutic time window for TH induction is currently unknown, it is prudent to initiate TH as quickly as feasible after ROSC.

Pearls of Care

1. Cellular damage from ischemia/reperfusion injury is a *dynamic process*, and a therapeutic window exists after resuscitation from cardiac arrest during which damage, especially neurological damage, can be attenuated.
2. Therapeutic hypothermia is the first proven therapy to improve neurological outcome after resuscitation from cardiac arrest, indicating that brain injury related to cardiac arrest is in fact a treatable condition.
3. Therapeutic hypothermia is indicated for patients who are not following commands after ROSC from VF cardiac arrest, and it should also be considered for patients with non-VF initial rhythms who are not following commands after ROSC.
4. Neurological prognostication is notoriously challenging in the first few days after resuscitation from cardiac arrest, and in most cases attempts at prognostication should be withheld until the 72-hour mark after ROSC.

Selected Readings

Arrich J, Holzer M, Herkner H, Müllner M. Hypothermia for neuroprotection in adults after cardiopulmonary resuscitation. *Cochrane Database of Systematic Reviews* 2009;4:CD004128.

Bernard SA, Gray TW, Buist MD, et al. Treatment of comatose survivors of out-of-hospital cardiac arrest with induced hypothermia. *N Engl J Med* 2002;346(8):557–563.

Hypothermia after Cardiac Arrest (HACA) Investigators. Mild therapeutic hypothermia to improve the neurologic outcome after cardiac arrest. *N Engl J Med* 2002;346(8):549–556.

Kilgannon JH, Jones AE, Shapiro NI, et al. Association between arterial hyperoxia following resuscitation from cardiac arrest and in-hospital mortality. *JAMA* 2010;303(21):2165–2171.

Negovsky VA. The second step in resuscitation—the treatment of the "post-resuscitation disease." *Resuscitation* 1972;1(1):1–7.

Neumar RW, Nolan JP, Adrie C, et al. Post-cardiac arrest syndrome: epidemiology, pathophysiology, treatment, and prognostication. A consensus statement from the International Liaison Committee on Resuscitation (American Heart Association,

Australian and New Zealand Council on Resuscitation, European Resuscitation Council, Heart and Stroke Foundation of Canada, InterAmerican Heart Foundation, Resuscitation Council of Asia, and the Resuscitation Council of Southern Africa); the American Heart Association Emergency Cardiovascular Care Committee; the Council on Cardiovascular Surgery and Anesthesia; the Council on Cardiopulmonary, Perioperative, and Critical Care; the Council on Clinical Cardiology; and the Stroke Council. *Circulation* 2008;118(23):2452–2483.

Peberdy MA, Callaway CW, Neumar RW, et al. Part 9: post-cardiac arrest care: 2010 American Heart Association Guidelines for Cardiopulmonary Resuscitation and Emergency Cardiovascular Care. *Circulation* 2010;122(18 Suppl 3):S768–786.

Trzeciak S, Jones AE, Kilgannon JH, et al. Significance of arterial hypotension after resuscitation from cardiac arrest. *Crit Care Med* 2009;37(11):2895–2903.

Young GB. Neurologic prognosis after cardiac arrest. *N Engl J Med* 2009;361(6):605–611.

Chapter 9

Intracranial Hemorrhage and Acute Ischemic Stroke

Opeolu Adeoye and Edward C. Jauch

Introduction

Stroke is a leading cause of death and disability, with an estimated 795,000 new or recurrent strokes occuring each year in the United States. Of these, 87% are acute ischemic strokes (AIS), 10% are intracerebral hemorrhages (ICH), and 3% are subarachnoid hemorrhages (SAH). While prevention is the cornerstone of minimizing the burden of stroke, appropriate early treatment of acute stroke may reverse ischemia, prevent further acute injury, and minimize secondary injury, thus reducing morbidity and mortality.

Definition of Terms

Infarction: the death or necrosis of an area of tissue
Ischemia: reduced blood flow and organ dysfunction secondary to vascular obstruction
Penumbra: potentially salvageable area of ischemic tissues adjacent to infarcted tissues
Stroke: sudden-onset neurological impairment secondary to ischemia of or hemorrhage into an area of the brain

Clinical Syndromes

Neurological impairment after AIS results from reduced blood flow to a region of the brain. Without early reperfusion, brain ischemia progresses to infarction and permanent disability within minutes to a few hours. Areas adjacent to the infarct core may survive for several hours if collateral flow is present. Secondary injury may be exacerbated by derangements in serum glucose, body temperature, blood pressure, or oxygen saturation; treating these can minimize secondary injury in both AIS and ICH.

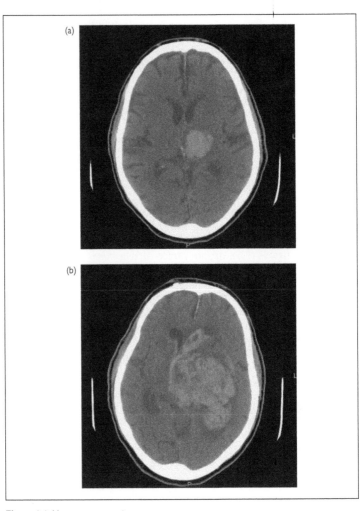

Figure 9.1 Hematoma expansion.

Spontaneous ICH occurs in an estimated 2 million people worldwide each year and has a 30-day mortality of 32%–50%. Hematoma expansion occurs in up to 40% of ICH patients within the first few hours, adding to morbidity and mortality (Fig. 9.1). Hematoma expansion is more common and fatal with ICH related to anticoagulation use. For this reason, minimizing or preventing hematoma expansion is an important therapeutic goal in ICH.

General and Key Management Controversies

Early emergency department (ED)–based interventions have three goals: (1) prevent enlargement of the areas affected by the stroke, (2) reverse injurious processes, for example by providing reperfusion in AIS, and (3) minimize secondary injury by optimizing physiologic conditions. All forms of stroke benefit from some common interventions while other interventions are type specific. The emergency physician plays a key role in the delivery of these therapies.

Early assessment of airway, breathing, and circulation (ABC) is essential, but few patients with ICH and even fewer with AIS require emergent intervention on arrival. Edema development and hematoma expansion may cause acute neurologic deterioration; thus, constant reassessment of the ABC is important.

In all forms of stroke, blood pressure (BP) assessment is important. In AIS, uncontrolled hypertension will prevent use of intravenous recombinant tissue plasminogen activator (rt-PA). Current guidelines require the eligible patients to have a BP less than 185 mm Hg systolic and 110 mm Hg diastolic. Titrated or continuous infusions of antihypertensive agents, commonly nicardipine, may be used to bring the BP to within appropriate levels. Agents that may be considered for BP control include labetalol, nicardipine, clevidipine, hydralazine, and esmolol (Table 9.1). Nitroprusside is best avoided in neurological emergencies due to its unreliable dose-response profile and is not appropriate for pre- rt-PA management. If the patient is not a candidate for rt-PA, more generous permissive hypertension is encouraged unless concomitant end-organ injury, such as acute myocardial infarction, congestive heart failure, or aortic dissection, requires BP reduction. Avoid aggressive reduction of BP and iatrogenic relative hypotension, outside of rt-PA or other reperfusion therapies in AIS, to minimize further reductions in brain perfusion.

Elevated BP at presentation occurs frequently in ICH and is associated with worse outcomes. However, early aggressive reduction in BP has been controversial since more rapid BP decline during the first 24 hours after ICH is associated with poor outcomes. Elevated BP may contribute to hematoma expansion, but aggressive BP reduction may compromise perihematomal blood flow and contribute to secondary injury after ICH.

The Intensive Blood Pressure Reduction in Acute Cerebral Haemorrhage Trial (INTERACT) randomized ICH patients diagnosed by computed tomography (CT) within 6 hours of symptom onset with elevated systolic BP (150–220 mm Hg) to intensive BP reduction (target systolic BP 140 mm Hg; n = 203) or standard guideline-based management of BP (target systolic BP 180 mm Hg; n = 201). The relative risk of hematoma expansion was 36% lower (95% CI 0–59%, p = 0.05) in the intensive group than in the guideline group, and intensive BP reduction did not impact the risks of adverse events or outcomes at 90 days. A confirmatory phase III trial, INTERACT2, is ongoing.

The AHA Guidelines for the Management of ICH recommend mean arterial pressure <130 mm Hg with cerebral perfusion pressure (CPP) maintained

Table 9.1 Common IV Antihypertensive Agents Used in Acute Stroke

Agent	Mechanism	Typical Starting Dose
Hydralazine	Direct acting smooth muscle relaxant	10–20 mg bolus
Labetalol	Non selective alpha and beta blocker (more potent beta blocker)	10–20 mg bolus, may repeat bolus—or— 10 mg bolus followed by continuous infusion 2–8 mg/hr
Esmolol	Beta1-selective adrenergic receptor blocker	80 mg loading dose over 30 s then 150 mcg/kg/min. 300 mcg/kg/min maximum maintenance dose.
Nicardipine	Calcium channel blocker	5 mg/hr and titrate by 2.5 mg/hr every 5–15 mins
Clevidipine	Calcium channel blocker	1–2 mg/h, double rate every 90 s initially, then titrate every 5–10 min once close to desired BP

>60 mm Hg in patients with elevated intracranial pressure (ICP). A goal mean arterial pressure of 110 mm Hg is recommended for patients without elevated ICP. Reduction of systolic BP to 140 mm Hg is thought to be safe in patients with a presenting systolic BP of 150–220 mm Hg.[1]

Hyperglycemia after stroke is common and associated with a worse clinical outcome, suggesting the need for acute glycemic control. Treatment should achieve euglycemia without inducing iatrogenic hypoglycemia, which also can worsen clinical outcomes. Exact thresholds for acute glycemic interventions are not know but recent guidelines recommend keeping serum glucose below 180 mg/dL.

Therapeutic hypothermia for patients suffering all forms of acute stroke is promising but data to date are equivocal. Hyperthermia—even slight—in the setting of acute stroke is clearly associated with poor clinical outcomes. Even modest hyperthermia should be treated and avoided.

Optimal oxygen therapy after stroke remains unclear. Avoid hypoxemia to prevent extension of the ischemic infarct. There is no clear benefit and there may be harm from supernormal oxygen levels, which could increase oxidative stress through the production of reactive oxygen species. Until further evidence clarifies the subject, current guidelines call for the administration of supplemental oxygen to maintain oxygen saturation above 94%.

Condition Specific Interventions—Acute Ischemic Stroke

Reperfusion therapies for AIS include a single intravenous fibrinolytic drug and several intra-arterial approaches for thrombectomy. When performed early enough, reperfusion can reverse the ischemic insult. Intravenous rt-PA remains the only approved medical therapy for ischemic stroke. The National Institute of Neurological Disorders and Stroke rt-PA stroke study demonstrated that patients treated with rt-PA within 3 hours of symptom onset were more likely to have minimal or no disability at 3 months compared with those treated with placebo. Subsequently, the European Cooperative Acute Stroke Study III showed that rt-PA administered to carefully selected patients in the 3–4.5 hour window also had improved clinical outcomes.[2] While symptomatic intracranial hemorrhage was more frequent in rt-PA treated patients in both studies, mortality was not increased.

Thus, guidelines recommend intravenous administration of rt-PA within 4.5 hours of symptom onset in carefully selected eligible patients. *The earlier an individual patient is treated, the more likely that patient is to benefit from rt-PA therapy.* The probability of a good clinical outcome decreases with increasing time to reperfusion.

To avoid presentations outside the time window during which patients are eligible for rt-PA, lay education, pre-hospital training, and ED management of acute stroke emphasize rapid recognition of stroke symptoms, emergency medical service transport to a stroke-ready hospital, rapid triage and evaluation in the ED, and prompt screening for rt-PA eligibility.[3,4] In patients who are eligible for rt-PA, treatment should occur within 1 hour of ED arrival. To achieve this goal, evaluation of the patient by the ED physician should evaluate the patient within 10 minutes of arrival, notify the stroke team within 15 minutes, obtain a head CT within 25 minutes, and interpret the CT within 45 minutes. Emergency medical service systems ideally will have preplanned destination hospitals able to meet these goals for patients with suspected acute stroke.

Endovascular treatments, alone or in combination with rt-PA, are a treatment option for AIS, especially for those caused by larger proximal artery occlusions. A recent meta-analysis noted that the current data supporting endovascular therapy for AIS are primarily from single-arm, noncomparative studies.[5] Recent guidelines recommend intra-arterial thrombolysis within 6 hours of symptom onset for patients with proven middle cerebral artery (MCA) occlusions who are not candidates for intravenous rt-PA. Patients with contraindications to systemic thrombolysis (e.g., recent surgery) but without a large vessel occlusion may also be considered for intra-arterial therapy. Intra-arterial therapy is discouraged as primary treatment in patients who are eligible for intravenous rt-PA. The ongoing phase III Interventional Management of Stroke III trial is comparing intravenous rt-PA alone to intravenous rt-PA plus endovascular therapy.

Malignant MCA territory infarction, a stroke which rapidly produces a large volume of irreversible ischemia with associated edema producing significant mass effect and herniation (Fig. 9.2), may occur in up to 10% of all ischemic strokes and has an associated mortality rate as high as 80%. Recent randomized clinical trials demonstrate better survival and functional outcome with decompressive hemicraniectomy within 48 hours of symptom onset compared with standard medical therapy in patients who are 60 or younger, with decreased

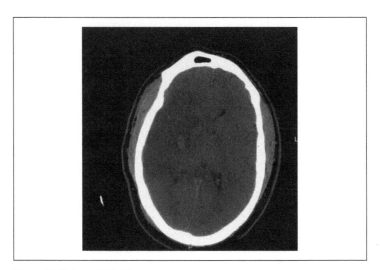

Figure 9.2 Malignant MCA Infarct.

level of consciousness, and with stroke volumes of greater than 145 mL by magnetic resonance imaging or greater than 50% of the MCA distribution by CT. Thus, younger patients with large hemispheric stroke should be managed at stroke centers with neurosurgical support for possible hemicraniectomy.

Surgical intervention is also lifesaving and promotes good outcomes in patients with cerebellar infarction. Delayed edema after cerebellar infarction sometimes leads to precipitous neurological deterioration and death. Patients with a suspected posterior circulation stroke should be monitored in a neurological intensive care unit and evaluated for potential surgical intervention. Decompressive surgical evacuation is recommended for patients with space occupying edema secondary to a cerebellar infarct.[3]

Condition Specific Interventions—Intracerebral Hemorrhage

Procoagulant drugs may reduce hematoma expansion but do not clearly improve clinical outcomes after ICH. The lack of overall benefit may be from increased numbers of patients with intraventricular hemorrhage (IVH) in one trial or the approximately 20% increase in arterial thrombotic complications after rFVIIa in another. Subgroup analyses suggest that younger patients with a baseline ICH volume less than 60 mL, minimal IVH, and presenting within 2.5 hours of symptom onset may benefit from rFVIIa.[6] The "spot sign" or contrast extravasation on CT angiography may also help identify ICH patients likely to experience hematoma expansion. Pending further studies, rFVIIa is not recommended for clinical use in ICH at this time.[1]

Anticoagulant-associated ICH (AAICH) accounts for 1 in 5 of all ICH cases, and coagulopathy results in larger hematomas, hematoma expansion, and mortality. Normalization of the International Normalized Ratio (INR) at 24 hours after AAICH is a direct result of how quickly fresh frozen plasma (FFP) is administered in the ED. Prothrombin complex concentrates (PCC) are an alternative or adjunct to FFP administration. Patients who receive PCC have faster times to correction of their INR and received less volume of FFP but clinical outcomes do not differ. Current guidelines recommend withholding warfarin and administering intravenous vitamin K and FFP or PCCs in patients with AAICH secondary to warfarin.

Condition Specific Interventions—Subarachnoid Hemorrhage

Careful attention to the ABCs is required in patients with aneurysmal SAH. No data to date have identified optimal targets for BP control; however, elevated BP can be managed with the same agents as previously recommended for ischemic and hemorrhagic stroke. Evidence of vasospasm typically is seen within 3 to 5 days from rupture. For the prevention of symptomatic vasospasm/delayed cerebral ischemia, oral nimodipine should be administered.

Pearls of Care

1. Early and ongoing physiologic optimization of oxygenation, BP, glucose, and temperature are key for all forms of stroke.
2. EDs should have systems in place for rapid evaluation of potential AIS that facilitate administration of intravenous rt-PA in eligible patients.
3. Endovascular procedures may be considered within 8 hours of symptom onset in ischemic stroke patients who are not eligible for IV rt-PA or who fail to respond to IV rt-PA.
4. Consider emergent transfer of patients with large hemispheric or cerebellar infarcts to centers where lifesaving neurosurgical interventions may be performed.
5. Patients on anticoagulant therapy should immediately receive corrective therapy in the ED, even if being transferred to another center.

References

1. Morgenstern LB, Hemphill JC, 3rd, Anderson C, et al. Guidelines for the management of spontaneous intracerebral hemorrhage: a guideline for healthcare professionals from the American Heart Association/American Stroke Association. *Stroke* 2010;41(9):2108–2129.

2. Hacke W, Kaste M, Bluhmki E, et al. Thrombolysis with alteplase 3 to 4.5 hours after acute ischemic stroke. *N Engl J Med* 2008;359(13):1317–1329.

3. Adams HP, Jr., del Zoppo G, Alberts MJ, et al. Guidelines for the early management of adults with ischemic stroke: a guideline from the American Heart Association/American Stroke Association Stroke Council, Clinical Cardiology Council, Cardiovascular Radiology and Intervention Council, and the Atherosclerotic Peripheral Vascular Disease and Quality of Care Outcomes in Research Interdisciplinary Working Groups: the American Academy of Neurology affirms the value of this guideline as an educational tool for neurologists. *Stroke* 2007;38(5):1655–1711.

4. Jauch EC, Cucchiara B, Adeoye O, et al. Part 11: adult stroke: 2010 American Heart Association Guidelines for Cardiopulmonary Resuscitation and Emergency Cardiovascular Care. *Circulation* 2010;122(18 Suppl 3):S818–S828.

5. Baker WL, Colby JA, Tongbram V, et al. Neurothrombectomy devices for the treatment of acute ischemic stroke: state of the evidence. *Ann Int Med* 2011;154(4):243–252.

6. Mayer SA, Davis SM, Skolnick BE, et al. Can a subset of intracerebral hemorrhage patients benefit from hemostatic therapy with recombinant activated factor VII? *Stroke* 2009;40(3):833–840.

Selected Readings

Adams HP, Jr., del Zoppo G, Alberts MJ, et al. Guidelines for the early management of adults with ischemic stroke: a guideline from the American Heart Association/American Stroke Association Stroke Council, Clinical Cardiology Council, Cardiovascular Radiology and Intervention Council, and the Atherosclerotic Peripheral Vascular Disease and Quality of Care Outcomes in Research Interdisciplinary Working Groups: the American Academy of Neurology affirms the value of this guideline as an educational tool for neurologists. *Stroke* 2007;38(5):1655–1711.

Arima H, Anderson CS, Wang JG, et al. Lower treatment blood pressure is associated with greatest reduction in hematoma growth after acute intracerebral hemorrhage. *Hypertension* 2010;56(5):852–858.

Khatri P, Abruzzo T, Yeatts SD, Nichols C, Broderick JP, Tomsick TA. Good clinical outcome after ischemic stroke with successful revascularization is time-dependent. *Neurology* 2009;73(13):1066–1072.

Mayer SA, Brun NC, Begtrup K, et al. Efficacy and safety of recombinant activated factor VII for acute intracerebral hemorrhage. *N Engl J Med* 2008;358(20):2127–2137.

Morgenstern LB, Hemphill JC, 3rd, Anderson C, et al. Guidelines for the management of spontaneous intracerebral hemorrhage: a guideline for healthcare professionals from the American Heart Association/American Stroke Association. *Stroke* 2010;41(9):2108–2129.

Chapter 10

Management of the Critically Poisoned Patient

Eric J. Lavonas

Introduction

Each day, nearly 2000 people are treated in US emergency departments (EDs) due to unintentional poisoning, with 22% being admitted for care.[1] Poisoning causes more than 40,000 deaths per year in the United States, more than double since 1999 and now exceeding those from motor vehicle crashes.[2]

Routine consultation with a regional poison center (1-800-222-1222) is recommended for all known or suspected poisonings, particularly when the illness is severe. However, telephonic advice is not a substitute for critical decision making at the bedside.

Definition of Terms

A *toxin* is a substance introduced into the human body that disrupts physiologic processes causing harm. This term is used synonymously with *poison*.

Clinical Syndromes

Critically ill patients may not provide an accurate history. In cases involving self-harm, overdose by multiple medications is common. It is important to obtain information from all available sources, including the family and friends, containers, pharmacy records, and medical records. With the exception of certain medications such as acetaminophen, salicylates, anticonvulsants, lithium, and digoxin, serum drug levels are rarely available in a time frame that supports early resuscitation decisions.

A "toxidrome" is a constellation of clinical signs, symptoms, and laboratory findings that suggests the effects of a specific toxin; recognition of a toxidrome can facilitate emergency stabilizing care and provide a targeted differential diagnosis. However, it is important to maintain a broad differential diagnosis, as natural disease can mimic the presentation of severe poisoning and vice versa.

General and Key Management Controversies

Care for poisoned patients should begin in a monitored treatment area, particularly when the history is uncertain. Hypotension, dysrhythmia, central nervous system (CNS) depression, hypoventilation, seizures, falls, elopement, and repeat self-harm attempts can occur without warning.

Patients with chemical contamination of their skin, hair, or clothing should be disrobed and cleaned, with care taken to avoid spreading contamination to staff or other patients.

Gastrointestinal decontamination, once a ubiquitous feature in the management of ingested toxins, now has a limited role. Gastric lavage and whole-bowel irrigation are rarely used, and syrup of ipecac is not available in the United States. A single dose of activated charcoal may be given orally or via nasogastric tube to patients who present within 1 hour of ingestion of a life-threatening poison for which no adequate antidote is available. Administration of charcoal beyond this 1-hour window may be indicated for some medications, such as enteric-coated medications and aspirin, that have delayed absorption. Multiple-dose activated charcoal may block delayed absorption or speed elimination of specific toxins.[3] Charcoal should not be administered for ingestion of caustic substances, metals, hydrocarbons, or benign ingestions.

Airway protection is paramount and may require endotracheal intubation. Elevation of the head of the bed is a simple and effective way to reduce the risk of aspiration.

Testing

Limited laboratory testing is appropriate for most poisoned patients. When the history of exposure is unclear or untrustworthy, screening with a basic serum chemistry panel (electrolytes, total CO_2, renal function, glucose), electrocardiogram (EKG), and serum acetaminophen level to identify the most life-threatening toxin-related processes should be performed. Women should receive a pregnancy test.

Beyond this short list, testing should be driven by specific elements in the history, physical examination, and other laboratory tests (e.g., to further work up metabolic acidosis).

Urine screening for drugs of abuse rarely changes medical management, but it may be useful information for the psychiatric consultant.[4]

A partial listing of medications used to treat life-threatening poisoning is provided in Table 10.1. In most cases, the optimal dose of these medications has not been determined. Consultation with a regional poison center or local expert, such as a medical toxicologist, is recommended when managing severely poisoned patients.

Agitated Delirium

Patients who present with psychomotor agitation, often accompanied by violent behavior, pose a unique set of challenges for the emergency physician.

Table 10.1 Partial List of Medications Used to Treat Life-Threatening Poisoning

Drug	Typical Uses	Adult Dose	Pediatric Dose	Notes
Activated charcoal (single dose)	Life-threatening ingestions presenting within 1 hour	50 g PO/NG	1 g/kg PO/NG	Protect airway if needed
Activated charcoal (multiple dose)	Carbamazepine Salicylates Theophylline	As above, then 25 g PO/NG Q1–2H	As above, then 0.5 g/kg PO/NG Q1–2H	Hold if no bowel sounds
Atropine	Carbamates Organophosphates	1 mg IV, double dose and repeat Q3minutes, no maximum	0.02 mg/kg IV, double dose and repeat Q3minutes, maximum dose unclear	Titrate to control of respiratory secretions and airway resistance
Calcium	Beta blockers Calcium channel blockers	1–2 g calcium chloride (10–20 mL of 10% solution) or 3–6 g calcium gluconate (30–60 mL of 10% solution) IV	20 mg/kg calcium chloride (0.2 mL/kg of 10% solution) or 60 mg/kg calcium gluconate (0.6 mL/kg) of 10% solution) IV	Calcium gluconate preferred in children and when using a peripheral IV. Repeat if needed. Hourly infusion rate same as bolus rate.
Digoxin immune Fab	Digoxin and related glycosides	Known ingestion: 1 vial IV per 500–600 mcg digoxin ingested Known serum level: dose (vials, IV) = digoxin level (ng/mL) x weight (kg)/100 Cardiovascular collapse (empiric therapy): 10–20 vials IV	Known ingestion: Same as adult Known serum level: Same as adult Cardiovascular collapse (empiric therapy): 3–6 vials	

(continued)

Table 10.1 (Continued)

Drug	Typical Uses	Adult Dose	Pediatric Dose	Notes
Ethanol	Ethylene glycol Methanol	Loading dose: 600 mg/kg (7.6 mL/kg of 10% solution) IV Maintenance IV infusion, nondrinker: Start at 66 mg/kg per hour (0.83 mL/kg per hour). Double maintenance infusion dose in chronic drinkers	Same as adult	Fomepizole is preferred Reduce or eliminate loading dose if serum ethanol is present Titrate to serum ethanol level 100–150 mg/kg Adjust dosing during dialysis Use of standard calculator (e.g., in Micromedex) strongly encouraged
Flumazenil	Benzodiazepines	0.2 mg (2 mL) IV Q1minute until reversal, max 3 mg	0.01 mL/kg (0.1 mL/kg) IV Q1minute until reversal, max 0.05 mg/kg	Avoid in polypharmacy ingestions and patients with a history of seizure
Folic acid	Methanol	50 mg IV Q4–6 hours	1 mg/kg IV Q4–6hours	May use folinic acid (leucovorin), same dose
Fomepizole	Ethylene glycol Methanol	15 mg/kg IV ×1, then 10 mg/kg IV Q12H	Same as adult	Adjust dosing during dialysis
Glucagon	Beta blocker Calcium channel blocker	3–10 mg IV bolus, then 3–5 mg/hr IV infusion	0.05–0.15 mg/kg IV bolus, then 0.05–0.10 mg/kg per hour IV infusion	Anticipate vomiting with loading dose
Hydroxocobalamin	Cyanide	5 g IV over 5–15 minutes Repeat in 15 minutes PRN	70 mg/kg IV over 5–15 minutes Repeat in 15 minutes PRN	May give with sodium thiosulfate (separate IV)
Lipid emulsion	Local anesthetics Beta blockers Calcium channel blockers Other drugs	1.5 mL/kg IV bolus, repeated Q3–5minutes PRN to max 3 mL/kg Follow with infusion, 0.25 mL/kg per minute IV for 30–60 minutes	Same as adult	20% solution of long-chain fatty acids (e.g., Intralipid®) most studied

		Adult	Pediatric	Comments
Insulin (high dose)	Beta blockers Calcium channel blockers	1–2 unit/kg IV bolus, given with 0.5 g/kg dextrose (1 mL/kg of D50 solution) Follow with infusion, 0.5–2 units/kg per hour IV, given with dextrose infusion (0.5 g/kg per hour, titrated to serum glucose 100–150 mg/dL)	Same as adult, except D10 or D25 solution preferred in smaller children	Check blood sugar and potassium frequently Give potassium to maintain serum potassium 2.5–2.8 mEq/L
Naloxone	Opioids	0.04–0.4 mg IV, repeat Q2–3minutes and escalate dose PRN to max 10 mg	0.1 mg/kg IV, repeat Q2–3 mins PRN	Titrate to reversal of respiratory depression and restoration of airway protection May also be given IM, IO, intralingual, intranasal, or endotracheal
Octreotide	Sulfonylureas	50–100 mcg, IV or SC	1 mcg/kg, IV or SC	Repeat dosing or infusion sometimes required
Pyridoxine	Isoniazid (INH)	5 g IV	70 mg/kg IV	Alternate:1 mg pyridoxine per mg INH ingested
Sodium bicarbonate	Cocaine Tricyclic antidepressants	50–75 mEq IV (50–75 mL of 8.4% solution), repeated Q3–5minutes PRN	1 mEq/kg IV (1 mL/kg of 8.4% solution), repeatedQ3–5minutes PRN	Check pH and sodium frequently. Dilute before administration in small children
Sodium nitrite	Cyanide	300 mg IV over 3–5 mins, repeat x1 PRN	10 mg/kg IV over 3–5 mins, repeat x1 PRN	Hydroxocobalamin preferred Reduce dose in patients with anemia
Sodium thiosulfate	Cyanide	12.5 g (50 mL of 25% solution) IV over 10 minutes, repeat x1 PRN	400 mg/kg (1.65 mL/kg of 25% solution) IV over 10 minutes	Usually given with hydroxocobalamin or sodium nitrite Use separate IV from hydroxocobalamin

IM, intramuscular; IV, intravenous.

This presentation can be caused by toxic ingestion, other medical disorders, psychiatric disorders, or any combination thereof.

Management of agitated patients should begin with an attempt at verbal de-escalation. An offer of food can be surprisingly effective.

If verbal techniques fail, the patient must be physically restrained safely. By controlling the limbs, shoulder girdle, and femoral crease area, struggling patients can be immobilized without applying pressure to the torso or abdomen. Immediately after physical control is achieved, finger-stick blood glucose measurement should be used to rule out hypoglycemia. Nonconstricting restraints should then be placed on all four limbs, and the patient should be placed supine on the stretcher.

Patients who continue to display psychomotor agitation or struggle against restraints will require chemical sedation. A common approach is to use lorazepam and/or haloperidol. Emergency department protocols should provide close monitoring, frequent restraint checks, hydration, food, and toileting assistance for restrained patients.

Agitated delirium is a medical emergency that carries with it a risk of sudden death. The differential diagnosis for agitated delirium is long and includes trauma, infections, hypoglycemia, severe stimulant drug intoxications, hyperthermia, and withdrawal syndromes. The workup for altered mental status is described in Chapter 7.

Obtundation/Central Nervous System Depression

Many substances can produce CNS depression. In general, these can be managed with supportive care, including intubation and mechanical ventilation. Identification of the specific substance involved is often impossible and rarely necessary.

Naloxone effectively reverses CNS and respiratory depression from opioids and may be effective for some other intoxications (e.g., clonidine) that act through the mu opioid receptor. Naloxone may be administered by almost any route, including intravenous (IV), intramuscular (IM), endotracheal, intranasal, and intralingual. When possible, apneic patients should receive assisted ventilation prior to naloxone administration.[5] Although naloxone administration is generally safe, the drug precipitates an acute withdrawal syndrome in opioid-dependent patients. Therefore, recent recommendations call for a much lower starting dose than was previously used.[6] Dose escalation, up to 10 mg total, is sometimes required. Unfortunately, it is unclear how long a patient needs to be observed following successful reversal of CNS/respiratory depression with naloxone. A brief period (2–3 hours) is probably appropriate for patients with morphine or heroin overdose, but longer periods (8–12 hours or more) may be necessary for patients with life-threatening overdose of a long-acting or sustained-release opioid. Patients who develop recrudescent respiratory depression during the observation period can receive repeat naloxone dosing, followed by a naloxone infusion dosed at two-thirds of the waking dose per hour. Naloxone does not have a role in the management of cardiac arrest.

Although flumazenil effectively reverses CNS and respiratory depression from benzodiazepine overdosage, controversy surrounds the empiric use of flumazenil in patients with undifferentiated coma. This is because benzodiazepines may confer some protection in patients with severe tricyclic antidepressant overdoses, and 2%–4% of undifferentiated overdose patients in clinical trials of flumazenil developed adverse effects (mostly seizures). Most experts restrict the use of flumazenil to patients who are known not to have a history of benzodiazepine dependence or polydrug intoxication. Pediatric single-drug overdose cases and patients requiring reversal of benzodiazepine-based procedural sedation are often candidates for flumazenil therapy, while adult intentional overdose patients are better treated with supportive care alone.

Seizures

Benzodiazepines are the mainstay of therapy for both toxin-induced and non-toxin-induced seizures. Patients whose seizures fail to respond to adequate doses of benzodiazepines should be treated with barbiturates or propofol. Phenytoin should be avoided because it is ineffective in several classes of toxin-induced seizures and may cause harm in the setting of theophylline or cyclic antidepressant overdosage.

Concurrent with control of seizures is a search for an underlying cause; in particular, causes of seizure that require specific therapy, rather than just supportive care, must be identified. The most common and easily detected of these is hypoglycemia, most frequently caused by insulin or sulfonylurea overdosage, which responds to IV dextrose.

Recurrent or refractory hypoglycemia from sulfonylurea overdosage responds to octreotide.

Patients known or suspected to have seizures due to isoniazid overdosage should also receive IV pyridoxine.

Several toxicants, including salicylates, ethylene glycol, methanol, and vitamin A, can cause cerebral edema which can result in seizures.

Seizures caused by acetylcholinesterase inhibitors, such as organophosphate and carbamate insecticides, are treated with atropine and benzodiazepines. In addition, pralidoxime chloride is given for organophosphate poisoning.

In addition to general care and benzodiazepines, patients who seize from tricyclic antidepressant or other sodium channel blocker drug overdosage should receive IV sodium bicarbonate.

Toxin-Induced Cardiac Dysrhythmias

Wide Complex Tachycardia

Sodium channel blocking toxicants such as cyclic antidepressants, class Ia and Ic antiarrhythmics (e.g., quinidine, flecainide, propafenone), and cocaine impair the propagation of cardiac action potentials. Clinically, this presents as a wide QRS complexes on EKG, usually in a right bundle branch morphology. Patients may have hypotension, ventricular tachycardia, ventricular fibrillation, high-order AV nodal blockade, or asystole.

Patients should immediately receive boluses of IV sodium bicarbonate, titrated to a QRS duration <120–140 msec. Extremes of alkalosis (pH >7.50–7.55) and hypernatremia (sodium >150–155 mmol/L) should be avoided if possible. Ventilator adjustment may be used in conjunction with sodium bicarbonate to control PCO_2 and titrate serum pH.

Bradycardia and Hypotension

Toxin-induced bradycardia should be treated if it is associated with hypotension or clinical evidence of poor perfusion. Some common causes of toxin-induced bradycardia include digoxin, beta-blockers, calcium channel blockers, and clonidine.

Digoxin and related cardiac glycosides such as oleander inhibit ATP-dependent sodium-potassium exchange in the cell wall. The result is hyperkalemia, decreased heart rate, and increased cardiac contractility. Patients with hemodynamically significant bradycardia, high-order AV nodal blockade (Mobitz II second-degree block or complete heart block), or hyperkalemia (K >5.0 mmol/L) in the setting of digoxin toxicity should receive digoxin Fab antibodies.

Beta blockers and calcium channel blockers cause hypotension through decreases in heart rate, contractility, and peripheral arterial tone. Several treatment approaches use different mechanisms to address the resulting cardiogenic shock. It is common for patients to require several modalities simultaneously. Because of the danger of irreversible shock caused by prolonged hypoperfusion, different treatment strategies should be added and titrated in rapid succession until the mean arterial pressure and measures of core perfusion (urine output, lactate, etc.) show a good response. Treatment approaches include administration of atropine, calcium, glucagon, high-dose insulin, or vasopressors such as norepinephrine. In cases refractory to those previously described, transvenous pacemaker placement and intravenous lipid emulsion therapy have been tried with variable success. As a last resort, mechanical support of circulation, such as that provided by an extracoroporeal bypass circuit, intraaortic balloon pump, or ventricular assist device, may be required.

Clonidine and other centrally acting alpha-2 agonists cause hypotension by decreasing sympathetic outflow. Clinical features include miosis, CNS depression, bradycardia, hypotension, and apnea. The CNS depression and apnea may or may not respond to naloxone. Because cardiac and peripheral arterial receptors are unaffected, bradycardia and hypotension readily respond to IV fluids, atropine, and low doses of vasopressors such as norepinephrine.

Metabolic Acidosis

In an ED critical care setting, virtually all cases of metabolic acidosis will be accompanied by an increased anion gap. The differential diagnosis of an increased anion gap metabolic acidosis can be further divided by measuring the serum lactate level.

Toxicants associated with an elevated serum lactate level include metformin, cyanide, iron, and occasionally carbon monoxide.

Toxicants that produce metabolic acidosis with a normal serum lactate level include ethylene glycol, methanol, salicylates, and ibuprofen. With the exception of ibuprofen, severe poisoning with each of these agents requires specific interventions beyond standard care.

Carbon monoxide poisoning rarely causes a lactic acidosis; an elevated serum lactate level in this setting should prompt a search for additional diagnoses, such as cyanide poisoning (e.g., from smoke inhalation), sepsis, or trauma. Because it may be neuroprotective, many US experts recommend that patients with significant carbon monoxide poisoning receive hyperbaric oxygen therapy.

Cyanide poisoning produces CNS depression and hypotension. Patients may be bradycardic or tachycardic. Serum lactic acid levels are a useful diagnosic tool and correlate with blood cyanide levels. The preferred treatment is hydroxocobalamin, given alone or with sodium thiosulfate. Alternately, the cyanide antidote kit (sodium nitrite plus sodium thiosulfate) may be used. High-flow oxygen should also be administered.

Ethylene glycol has minimal inherent toxicity until it is metabolized through alcohol dehydrogenase to glycolic acid and oxalic acid. Accumulation of these acids causes metabolic acidosis and renal failure. Treatment includes blockade of alcohol dehydrogenase with fomepizole or ethanol, followed by hemodialysis.

Methanol is more intoxicating than ethyl alcohol. Like ethylene glycol, methanol is metabolized via alcohol dehydrogenase to toxic metabolites, formaldehyde and formic acid. Accumulation of these acids causes metabolic acidosis and irreversible blindness. Treatment includes blockade of alcohol dehydrogenase (see earlier), folic acid, and hemodialysis.

Metformin overdosage produces profound lactic acidosis. Both metformin and lactic acid are readily dialyzable, and early initiation of hemodialysis speeds resolution in severe poisoning.

Salicylates cause nausea, vomiting, tinnitus, and diaphoresis. As toxicity increases, patients develop a central respiratory alkalosis, followed by metabolic acidosis. Maximum toxicity is often delayed because of prolonged absorption of salicylates in overdose.

Treatment includes replacement of intravascular volume with IV crystalloids, prevention of ongoing absorption with multiple doses of activated charcoal, and alkaline diuresis (150 mEq sodium bicarbonate plus 40 mEq KCl per liter of D5W, infused IV at 2x maintenance rate). Patients with uncompensated or severe metabolic acidosis, altered mental status, cerebral edema, pulmonary edema, or very high salicylate levels (>80–100 mg/dL) should receive hemodialysis.

Local Anesthetic Toxicity

Inadvertent IV administration of bupivacaine, mepivicaine, or lidocaine can cause seizures and cardiovascular collapse that are refractory to standard therapies. In this setting, rapid administration of IV lipid emulsion may be life-saving. This literature is evolving rapidly; a ready reference is maintained at http://www.lipidrescue.org.

Cocaine Toxicity

Acute cocaine intoxication causes tachycardia, chest pain, hypertension, diaphoresis, seizures, and hyperthermia. The mainstays of therapy are benzodiazepines, nitrates, and opioids. In specific cases, alpha antagonists (e.g., phentolamine for profound hypertension) or calcium channel blockers (e.g., verapamil for tachycardia with or without hypertension) may be used.

Wide complex dysrhythmias should be treated with IV sodium bicarbonate. Beta blockers should not be used in cocaine toxicity because of conflicting data about safety.

Pearls of Care

1. Start care for poisoned patients in a monitored treatment area.
2. Use empiric naloxone only in patients with respiratory depression, starting with a low dose (0.04–0.4 mg) titrated as needed.
3. Agitated delirium is a high-risk medical emergency.
4. In the hypotensive poisoned patient, rapidly add and titrate treatments.
5. Intravenous lipids are a new antidote that may be life-saving for certain poisonings.

References

1. Centers for Disease Control and Prevention. CDC issue brief: unintentional drug poisoning in the United States. Atlanta, GA: National Center for Injury Prevention and Control, Centers for Disease Control and Prevention, 2010.

2. Statistical abstract of the United States: 2011. Washington, DC: US Census Bureau, 2011. Available at: http://www.census.gov/compendia/statab/2011/tables/11s1102.pdf. [accessed on April 4, 2011].

3. American Academy of Clinical Toxicology and European Association of Poisons Centres and Clinical Toxicologists position statement and practice guidelines on the use of multi-dose activated charcoal in the treatment of acute poisoning. *J Toxicol Clin Toxicol* 1999;37:731–751.

4. Eldridge DL, Holstege CP. Utilizing the laboratory in the poisoned patient. *Clin Lab Med* 2006;26(1):13–30.

5. Morrison LJ, Deakin CD, Morley PT, et. al.. Part 8: Advanced life support: 2010 International consensus on cardiopulmonary resuscitation and emergency cardiovascular care science with treatment recommendations. *Circulation* 2010;122(suppl_2):S345–S421.

6. Vanden Hoek TL, Morrison LJ, Shuster M, et. al.. Part 12: Cardiac Arrest in Special Situations: 2010 American Heart Association Guidelines for Cardiopulmonary Resuscitation and Emergency Cardiovascular Care. *Circulation* 2010;122(suppl_3):S829–S861.

7. Selected ReadingsCenters for Disease Control and Prevention. CDC's issue brief: unintentional drug poisoning in the United States. 2010. Available at: http://www.cdc.gov/HomeandRecreationalSafety/pdf/poison-issue-brief.pdf. [accessed on April 5, 2011].

8. Engebretsen KM, Kaczmarek KM, Morgan J, Holger JS. High-dose insulin therapy in beta-blocker and calcium channel-blocker poisoning. *Clin Toxicol* 2011;49(4):277–283.

9. Jamaty C, Bailey B, Larocque A, Notebaert E, Sanogo K, Chauny J-M. Lipid emulsions in the treatment of acute poisoning: a systematic review of human and animal studies. *Clin Toxicol* 2019;48(1):1–27.

10. Morrison LJ, Deakin CD, Morley PT, et al. Part 8: Advanced life support: 2010 international consensus on cardiopulmonary resuscitation and emergency cardiovascular care science with treatment recommendations. *Circulation* 2010;122(suppl_2):S345–S421.

11. Murray DB, Bateman DN. Use of intravenous lipids. Not yet in all overdoses with failed resuscitation. *BMJ* 2011;242:d2265

12. Pollanen MS, Chiasson DA, Cairns JT, et al. Unexpected death related to restraint for excited delirium: a retrospective study of deaths in police custody and in the community. *CMAJ* 1998 ;158:1603–1607.

13. Vanden Hoek TL, Morrison LJ, Shuster M, et al. Part 12: Cardiac arrest in special situations: 2010 American Heart Association Guidelines for Cardiopulmonary Resuscitation and Emergency Cardiovascular Care. *Circulation* 2010;122(suppl_3):S829–S861.

Chapter 11

Multisystem Trauma and Burns

Raquel Forsythe

Introduction

Trauma is the leading cause of death in the United States for people under 45 years old and a major cause of morbidity and long-term disability. In addition, trauma accounts for approximately one-third of all intensive care unit (ICU) admissions. Most deaths after trauma occur in the first 4–6 hours after the injury. While deaths at the scene are best addressed with injury prevention efforts, the remainder of the early deaths are generally from exsanguinating hemorrhage and other potentially preventable causes. The latter includes injuries identified and addressed in the primary survey, including tension pneumothorax and airway obstruction. Advances in trauma care developed during the military conflicts in Iraq and Afghanistan have changed resuscitation and early critical care of injured patients.

The concept of damage control previously referred to operative surgical management, has now extended to the resuscitation of trauma patients who require a massive transfusion (MT). This damage control resuscitation (DCR) should begin upon presentation to the emergency department (ED). Some severely injured trauma patients develop a dilutional coagulopathy that is difficult to control. However, recent studies have noted that up to 25% of severely injured patients present with coagulopathy prior to significant fluid resuscitation. This early coagulopathy is associated with increased mortality. Thus, prevention, early identification and treatment of coagulopathy are key factors in hemostatic resuscitation.

Burns also represent a public health problem, with more than 1 million Americans seeking medical attention for burn wounds annually. Approximately 50,000 will require hospital admission and 4500 will die from thermal injury. Proper early management for severely burned patients begins with airway assessment for adequate oxygenation and ventilation. It is important to recognize any inhalation injury of the airway. Adequate fluid resuscitation is necessary to prevent the development of burn shock.

This chapter discusses the resuscitative aspects of trauma care, not specific injuries or approaches to diagnosis or therapy outside of these core principles.

Definition of Terms

Damage control: an effort to curtail loss or damage. It was a Merchant Marine term used to describe how to rescue a crew and vessel aboard a damaged ship. In the early 1990s, this concept was applied to trauma patients with surgical care focused on an initial abbreviated operation that focused on the cessation of hemorrhage and control of intraabdominal contamination. After appropriate resuscitation, the injuries are more definitively repaired.

Damage control resuscitation: an overall guiding concept for resuscitation that uses the concept of permissive hypotension (that is, not seeking "normal vital signs" as an endpoint initially but rather 90–100 mm Hg systolic pressure), rapid cessation of surgical bleeding, and hemostatic resuscitation.

Hemostatic resuscitation: advocates for resuscitation with fixed ratios of packed red blood cells (PRBCs), fresh frozen plasma (FFP), and platelets in a 1:1:1 ratio to minimize dilutional coagulopathy. The use of thawed plasma is encouraged to achieve this ratio from the time of admission to the ED. The use of crystalloid for patients with hemorrhagic shock is discouraged.

Massive transfusion (MT): the transfusion of 10 or more PRBCs in a 24-hour period.

Trauma-associated coagulopathy (TAC): a hypocoaguable state that occurs in severely injured patients. Multiple factors appear to contribute and the exact mechanisms remain to be elucidated. However, tissue hypoperfusion may lead to increased protein C activity that contributes to anticoagulation and hyperfibinolysis.

Thromboelastography (TEG): a laboratory method that may facilitate goal-directed hemostatic resuscitation. New rapid TEG studies can be done at the point of care and qualitatively measure coagulation status.

Clinical Syndromes

Blunt and Penetrating Trauma Core Syndromes

Initial management of critically injured trauma patients must include an assessment of injuries, the presence of active hemorrhage, the depth and severity of shock, and evidence of coagulopathy. Since multiple injuries are common, avoiding hypotension and hypoxemia is crucial to avoid secondary injury if traumatic brain injury (TBI) exists. In the ED, the goal is airway stabilization, shock therapy or prevention, and a rapid evaluation of multiply injured patients to allow an appropriate disposition to the operating room, angiography, or ICU. For the patient with active hemorrhage, the concept of DCR plays a key role until bleeding is stopped.

In the 1980s, the concept of the "bloody, vicious cycle" in trauma emerged. This led to the concept of damage control surgery. Initially used in the abdomen, with packing of severe hepatic injuries, control of intraabdominal hemorrhage and gastrointestinal tract contamination, it soon spread to other injuries.

Extension in to the thoracic cavity and damage control neurosurgery and ortho-pedics soon emerged. The concept of damage control is that it is "easier to stay out of trouble than to get out of trouble." Abbreviated operations attempt to avoid the physiologic derangements that ensue with long operative times, worsening hemodilution, and hypothermia.

The military experience has found that up to 15%–20% of deaths from trauma are potentially preventable mostly due to hemorrhage. A retrospective analysis of massively transfused soldiers found a striking difference in mortality depending upon the ratio of plasma to PRBCs transfused. Those transfused with a low ratio (1:8) of plasma to PRBCs had a mortality of 65%, while the high ratio (1:1.4) had a mortality of 19%. An intermediate group with a ratio of 1:2.5 had a mortality of 34%. The limitation to this retrospective analysis is the potential for survivorship bias: because plasma may have been administered after PRBCs, some patients bleed to death too quickly to achieve a low ratio, rather than surviving because of the low ratio. However, additional studies of both military and civilian injuries found that massively transfused patients with higher ratios of plasma to FFP have lower mortality. These data led to the institution of a military protocol with a goal to transfuse plasma: PRBCs in a 1:1 ratio.

Most major trauma centers have instituted massive transfusion protocols (MTPs). These protocols allow for preplanning with the Blood Bank for the rapid delivery of the large amounts of blood, plasma, and platelets that are required for patients with traumatic hemorrhage.

In the ED, activation of the MTP that includes the use of thawed plasma can help to immediately begin addressing resuscitation coagulopathy. DCR starts with identification of patients at high risk for requiring MT. Prediction equations for MT have been developed for both military and civilian trauma patients who have predominantly penetrating and blunt injuries, respectively. These models typically include blood pressure, heart rate, base deficit, INR, hemoglobin, and presence of intraabdominal fluid on FAST exam.

Once identified, bleeding should be controlled as rapidly as possible. This may require operative intervention or angiography. Throughout the resuscitation, starting in the ED, limit crystalloid use to avoid hemodilution and worsening coagulopathy. Also, prevent hypothermia with active and passive warming. MT incites hypocalcemia; monitor and treat based on the ionized calcium levels.

Another recent addition to the treatment of traumatic coagulopathy is the use of the antifibrinolytic agent tranexemic acid. A recent multinational, randomized, prospective, placebo-controlled trial showed a decrease in mortality in trauma patients with active bleeding or at high risk for active bleeding. There was no increase in vascular occlusive events between the two groups of patients. The inclusion criteria for this study were simple and broad. Any patient with evidence of bleeding, systolic blood pressure less than 90 mm Hg, or tachycardia ≥110 beats per minute was enrolled. Tranexamic acid can be given up to 8 hours after injury, but it should be started as soon as bleeding is identified.

Thromboelastography (TEG) allows for goal-directed transfusion practices. TEG assesses clotting formation from the initial formation through breakdown of the clot. TEG provides a functional measure of the time to develop clot and the overall strength of the clot, and it is the only modality that demonstrates both thrombosis and lysis. The development of rapid-TEG machines that can quickly deliver point-of-care testing in the ED, OR, and ICU allows broader use of this modality. The main difference between standard and rapid TEG is the addition of tissue factor, resulting in a more rapid reaction and subsequent analysis. Early studies using rapid-TEG compared to conventional coagulation studies demonstrate the potential for a theoretical decrease in plasma transfusion.

Neurogenic Shock

When a cervical or upper thoracic cord lesion exists, hypotension (often without appropriate tachycardia) can result from loss of vasomotor tone. Hypotension after trauma is first presumed a volume deficit; if para- or quadriplegia accompanies the evaluation, or a bony disruption of the thoracic or cervical column is seen in an unresponsive patient, administer a vasopressor (norepinephrine, neosynephrine, or dopamine via titrated infusion) *after volume infusions* to restore perfusion and reverse shock.

Burns

Thermal injury evokes an inflammatory response that is proportional to the size and depth of the burn wound. In the initial 24–48 hours after a thermal injury, there is a breakdown in the integrity of the capillary membrane, resulting in a leak of the plasma volume into the interstitial space. This loss of capillary membrane integrity combined with an initial decrease in the cardiac output will lead to fatal burn shock if untreated. With proper fluid administration, shock is prevented and the patient will then develop a hypermetabolic response.

The assessment of any burn patient begins with the airway (see Chapter 15). Immediate intubation is required for those that are unconscious, in obvious respiratory distress, or with hemodynamic instability. Suspect inhalation injury in any patient with a history of smoke exposure in a closed space. Additional "hard signs" of impending airway obstruction include dyspnea, chest tightness, tachypnea, stridor, accessory muscle use, and swelling of the tongue and oropharynx. As a rule, early intubation is preferred to prevent later uncontrolled airway obstruction necessitating an emergent surgical airway. Bronchoscopy can aid assessment of the trachea and branches for airway injury. The upper airway is generally subject to thermal burns while the lower airway is at risk for chemical injury. Arterial blood gas analysis allows assessment carbon monoxide (CO) or other inhalation toxin poisoning. Do not rely on pulse oximetry, as the readings may be inaccurate. Treatment of CO poisoning is with 100% oxygen until carboxyhemoglobin levels fall below 10%, reserving hyperbaric oxygen treatments for those not in need of immediate surgery, hemodynamically stable, *and* with clear end-organ dysfunction (altered sensorium and ischemic chest pain are two common features).

The ideal fluid and formula for resuscitation of thermally injured is debated. In the initial phase, crystalloid remains the most common resuscitation fluid. Calculated volumes are given initially to restore perfusion with the goal of avoiding excessive fluid. Adverse consequences of fluid administration include pulmonary edema, pleural effusion, and the development of extremity and abdominal compartment syndromes.

To guide therapy, calculate the total body surface area (TBSA) of partial or full thickness burn. The "Rule of Nines" estimates the size of a burn in adults. In adults, anatomical regions represent 9% TBSA or a multiple thereof: head, neck, and each arm count as 9%, while the anterior trunk, posterior trunk, and individual legs are 18% each. For children, given the larger head size relative to the body, the Lund and Browder chart offers a more precise age-adjusted estimate.

An initial estimate of the fluid needs in a burn patient is best calculated using the Parkland formula. The total volume of fluid to be administered is calculated by multiplying 4 mL lactated Ringer's solution per kilogram of body weight by the percentage of total body surface area burn. Give half of the total calculated volume in the first 8 hours and deliver the remainder over the next 16 hours. This is an estimate of patient needs and *fluids must be adjusted* based on blood pressure and urine output, the latter measured hourly with an indwelling catheter. In adults, the goal is a urinary output of 0.5 to 1.0 mL/kg per hour. Children require 1.0 to 1.5 mL/kg per hour urinary output.

Patients with major medical comorbidities, including cardiac or renal disease, benefit from central monitoring of volume status. In most patients, two large-bore peripheral intravenous lines through nonburned skin are preferable for access.

Key Management Principles

Damage Control Resuscitation

- Rapid identification of patients at highest risk for the need for massive transfusion and to develop acute traumatic coagulopathy
- Permissive hypotension (targeting systolic blood pressure of 90 mm Hg) until bleeding is controlled
- Rapid control of hemorrhage (surgery, angiography)
- Prevention and treatment of hypothermia, acidosis, and hypocalcemia
- Minimize crystalloids to avoid hemodilution
- Early transfusion of blood products with high ratios of plasma and platelets to PRBCs
- Use of TEG to guide blood product administration

Use of Tranexamic Acid (CRASH-2 Study)

- Administer early and within 8 hours of injury for patients with active hemorrhage

- Dosage is a 1 gram loading dose over 10 minutes followed by an 8-hour maintenance infusion of 1 gram

Parkland Formula

- First 24 hours: 4 mL/kg per percent TSBA. Fluid of choice is lactated Ringer's solution. Administer half the volume in the first 8 hours and the rest over the next 16 hours (adults).

Pearls of Care

1. Trauma patients require a rapid assessment focused on seeking hemorrhage, neurologic injury, and potential need for massive transfusion.
2. Early initiation of massive transfusion protocols with high ratios of plasma and platelets to PRBCs decreases mortality in trauma patients.
3. Severely injured trauma patients may develop coagulopathy very early after injury. Use damage control resuscitation principles starting in the ED.
4. Thromboelastography aids in assessing functional coagulation status in severely injured patients and directing transfusion.
5. Initial resuscitation of burn patients must be based on TBSA burned and body mass, then adjusted to maintain urine flow and prevent the burn shock.

Selected Readings

Borgman MA, Spinella PC, Perkins JG, et al. Ratio of blood products transfused affects mortality in patients receiving massive transfusions at a combat support hospital. *J Trauma* 2007;63(4):805–813.

CRASH-2 trial collaborators, Shakur H, Roberts I, et al. Effects of tranexamic acid on death, vascular occlusive events, and blood transfusion in trauma patients with significant haemorrhage (CRASH-2): a randomised, placebo-controlled trial. *Lancet* 2010;376(9734):22–32.

Chapter 12

Massive Bleeding, Including Gastrointestinal Bleeding

Charles R. Wira III and Khoshal Latifzai

Introduction

Massive nontraumatic hemorrhage is a life-threatening condition creating hemo-dynamic instability, shock, or multisystem organ failure. Early identification, aggressive resuscitative care, and control of bleeding are mandatory for survival. The most common cause encountered in the emergency department (ED) is upper or lower gastrointestinal hemorrhage, but other causes include ruptured abdominal aortic aneurysm, ruptured ectopic pregnancy, spontaneous or iatro-genic retroperitoneal hemorrhage, spontaneous bleeding from malignancies, or spontaneous bleeding from an arterio-venous fistula. Localization of the source of bleeding is integral to eventual management.

Definition of Terms

Major hemorrhage is bleeding resulting in shock and hemodynamic instability. Some patients may present with compensated shock and a near normal blood pressure (systolic blood pressure [SBP] 90 mmHg or above or mean arterial pressure [MAP] 65 mm Hg or above), though closer inspection will suggest shock. One way to do this closer inspection is through the *Shock Index* (heart rate/systolic blood pressure). This index can quantify compensated shock pres-ence absent overt hypotension. Any Shock Index greater than 0.8 identifies compensated shock and is a predictor of later hypotension, transfusion require-ment, and cardiovascular collapse. An elevated blood lactate may also suggest occult shock despite a seemingly normal blood pressure.

The *shock severity grading system* utilized for traumatic hemorrhage is another instrument to aid in assessing blood loss (see Table 12.1). It must be considered in conjunction with the patient's source of bleeding and underlying comorbidi-ties because each may affect the clinical presentation and response to therapies. *Class 1 Shock* results from roughly 15% of blood loss (<750cc) and is associ-ated with a mild resting tachycardia. Geriatric patients or patients on negative chronotropic cardiac medications may have a blunted tachycardic response.

Table 12.1 Classifications of Hemorrhagic Shock

Class of Shock	Blood Loss (%)	Blood Volume Lost (cc)	Clinical Features
1	<15	<750	Mild resting tachycardia
2	15–30	750–1500	Moderate tachycardia, narrow pulse pressure, delayed capillary refill
3	30–40	1500–2000	Hypotension, end-organ hypoperfusion, oliguria, altered mentation
4	>40	>2000	Persistent hypotension, organ failure

Source: Adapted from American College of Surgeons Committee on Trauma. Shock. In: *Advanced trauma life support for doctors.* 7th ed. First Impression Press; 2004:74.

Class 2 Shock results from 15% to 30% blood loss (750–1500cc), manifesting a moderate tachycardia, narrow pulse pressure, and delayed capillary refill. *Class 3 Shock* is from 30% to 40% blood loss (1500–2000cc). The body's capacity to prevent hypotension is overwhelmed, and clinical signs of end-organ hypoperfusion begin to surface. The patient may become oliguric or develop a change in mental status. *Class 4 Shock* results from loss of more than 40% of the total blood volume (>2000cc) and is associated with persistent hypotension, multisystem organ failure, and potentially death.[1]

Multisystem organ failure can occur from massive bleeding secondary to global tissue hypoxia and the release of cytopathic inflammatory mediators. Markers of organ failure or hypoperfusion include clinical or serological signs of acute kidney injury, severe hypoxia, hepatic failure, altered mental status, cardiac biomarker elevations, an abnormal base deficit, or disseminated intravascular coagulation.

The most common form of massive bleeding is gastrointestinal hemorrhage, broadly divided into two types. *Upper gastrointestinal bleeds (UGIBs)* have a source between the proximal esophagus and the ligament of Treitz at the duodenojejunal flexure of the small intestine. *Lower gastrointestinal bleeds (LGIBs)* originate distal to this point.

Clinical Syndromes

Upper Gastrointestinal Bleeding

UGIBs account for roughly 100,000 hospital admissions annually, with peptic ulcer disease being the most common cause. Overall mortality from UGIB is about 10%,[2,3] and factors that decrease survival include age >60 years old, severe comorbidities, sustained active bleeding, hypotension, large transfusion requirements, and severe coagulopathy. Several clinical symptoms may localize the source of the bleed, including hematemesis, coffee-ground emesis, or the presences of melena. While bright red blood per rectum is usually from lower bleeding, it can occur in a rapid, high-volume UGIB. The physical exam should be comprehensive, including a digital rectal exam and abdominal exam.

There are two broad categories of acute UGIB: variceal and nonvariceal. Because this classification has different care implications, initial evaluation should aim to classify the presentation into one of these two groups. Clinical indicators of a variceal source of UGIB include a prior history of varices, underlying cirrhosis of the liver, and secondary physical exam findings suggesting severe liver disease (e.g., ascites, caput medusa, telangectasias, Muehrcke's lines in the fingernail, gynecomastia, or hypogonadism). Conversely, patients with nonvariceal UGIBs may have other predisposing causes such as nonsteroidal anti-inflammatory use.

Variceal bleeds account for 10%–30% of all UGIBs and occur in about half of those with cirrhosis.[4]These tend to be brisk given the high portal pressure. Of the remaining 90% of UGIBs, peptic ulcer disease and erosions account for the vast majority. Esophagitis and Mallory-Weiss tears are less common, while angiodysplasia, cancer, Dieulafoy lesions, and portal gastropathy are the least frequent.

Lower Gastrointestinal Bleeding

In Westernized countries, LGIBs account for roughly 25% of all cases of gastrointestinal hemorrhage. LGIBs have a slightly higher mortality range, approaching 10%–20%, compared to UGIB.[5,6] Clinical clues that favor the lower gastrointestinal tract as being the source of bleeding include the passage of maroon-colored stool or bright red blood per rectum.

LGIBs may be categorized into those originating from the colon and those from the small bowel. Colonic sources of LGIB include diverticular disease (30%–60% of LGIBs), angiodysplasia, cancer, post-procedural (e.g., post-polypectomy) bleeding, and colitis (inflammatory, infectious, or ischemic). Less common etiologies include colopathy due to radiation and aortoenteric fistulas. Small-bowel foci of LGIBs may include angiodysplasia, cancer, enteritis (inflammatory, infectious, or post-radiation), Meckel's diverticulum, and rarely, aortoenteric fistula.

Although resuscitation of a patient with a massive gastrointestinal bleed takes precedence over localization during the initial presentation, a few historical clues can be very helpful in localizing the source of the blood loss. These include items such as a history of a coagulopathy, anticoagulation medications, diverticular disease, or inflammatory bowel disease.

Other Causes of Major Medical Hemorrhage

Ruptured abdominal aortic aneurysms typically present with abdominal or back pain, often with syncope. Mortality rate approaches 60%–90% and is reduced to roughly 50% if patients are able to present to a hospital without evidence of shock.[7] Only half of patients have abdominal pulsations on physical exam, and definitive diagnosis is made by ultrasound or computed tomography (CT). Surgery is mandatory and should not be delayed by trying to restore blood pressure; hemorrhage control is the best option to improve survival.

Ectopic pregnancy needs to be entertained in the differential diagnosis for all females of child-bearing age who are pregnant and have amenorrhea, pelvic pain, abdominal pain, or vaginal bleeding, especially with syncope or hypotension. The absence of an intrauterine pregnancy in combination with a positive urine pregnancy test and evidence of free fluid in the abdomen by ultrasound can make the diagnosis, which requires resuscitation and surgical evaluation.

Retroperitoneal hemorrhage may be spontaneous or iatrogenic. Diagnosis can be made by a noncontrast enhanced CT of the abdomen and pelvis, reserving contrast for selected cases of smaller volume extravasation. Angiographic embolization can provide definitive cessation of bleeding.

General and Key Management and Controversies

Initial Resuscitation of the Bleeding Patient

Initial care of the patient with massive medical hemorrhage should consist of a primary survey assessing airway, breathing, and circulation. Patients with massive bleeding from an UGIB may need intubation to prevent aspiration. Visible hemorrhage (e.g., hemorrhage from an ulcerated hemodialysis fistula) should be controlled with direct pressure. To enable rapid infusion, at least two large-bore (14- to 16-gauge or larger) peripheral venous catheters and/or an 8.5 French central venous catheter should be placed. To enhance volume infusion, pressure bags and a mechanical rapid transfusion device may be employed. To mitigate the effects of hypothermia (e.g., coagulopathy) induced from the bleeding and the resuscitation, warmed crystalloid solutions (i.e., 0.9% normal saline or lactated Ringer's solution) can be used as initial volume expanders. Hypotensive patients should receive 500–1000 cc boluses rapidly and repeatedly until a mean arterial pressure of 60–65 mmHg, SBP of 90 mmHg, or a Shock Index of <0.8 is achieved to restore systemic perfusion to critical organs.

Following initial crystalloid fluid resuscitation, patients generally fall into one of three categories. Rapid responders become hemodynamically stable following crystalloid administration. Transient responders initially stabilize but then show signs of recurrent hypotension (SBP<90mmHg), while nonresponders do not stabilize despite aggressive resuscitation efforts. For acute providers managing patients with massive bleeding, transfusions should be guided by vital signs and clear blood loss rather than by the hemoglobin level. Transfusion of pRBCs should be administered immediately to transient responders (SBP<90mmHg after crystalloid) or nonresponders (SBP<90mmHg in spite of crystalloid) in addition to consideration of other emergent procedures (e.g., surgery).

Treatment for Upper Gastrointestinal Bleeding

As the patient is being resuscitated with fluids or blood products, pharmacologic therapy should be initiated. The choice of agent(s) depends on the type of bleed suspected (variceal vs. nonvariceal).In the undifferentiated patient, start with medications for both etiologies.

For presumed gastric bleeding, high-dose parenteral proton pump inhibitors (PPIs) protect the thrombus from fibrinolysis by maintaining the pH near a bleeding ulcer above 6.0. Pantoprazole, lansoprazole, and esomeprazole are available in intravenous form. For patients with presumed variceal hemorrhage, octreotide infusions lower pressure in the splanchnic and portal venous circulation and limit exsanguination from varices in these vessels.

Nasogastric lavage can aid in localization of the bleeding source, but it is often poorly tolerated and is an insensitive test or therapy. Caution should be employed in patients with coagulopathies because nasogastric tube placement could cause massive epistaxis. By virtue of its ability to directly visualize the source of bleeding, endoscopy plays both a diagnostic and therapeutic role in the management of UGIB. Because 10% of hemodynamically unstable patients with hematochezia actually have an upper gastrointestinal source of bleeding, urgent upper endoscopy merits consideration in this patient population.[8]Variceal hemorrhage can be controlled endoscopically using thermal cautery, slerotherapy, band ligation, or glue injection. Nonvariceal hemorrhage can be controlled endoscopically using epinephrine injection, thermal cautery, bi- or monopolar cautery, hemoclip deployment, or sclerosant injections.

If endoscopy is not readily available, bleeding can be temporized using a Sengstaken-Blakemore or similar tube to tamponade the vessels. If hemorrhage causes persistent hypotension or is refractory to the aforementioned measures, angiographic embolization or surgery is an alternative strategy.

Treatment for Lower Gastrointestinal Bleeding

In well-resuscitated patients without ongoing brisk bleeding, colonoscopy may be performed to determine the source of as well as to treat an LGIB. Therapeutic options during colonoscopy include coagulation, injection with sclerosing or vasoconstrictor agents, or other endoscopically guided procedures.

For hemodynamically stable patients with evidence of ongoing bleeding, a radionuclide tagged red blood cell (RBC) scan may be performed for localization of bleeding. Reliability is compromised with slower bleeding rates, with only 45%–55% of those performed being able to accurately localize bleeding in the clinical setting.[9] For stable patients, the next option is angiography, which can be diagnostic and therapeutic. Therapeutic interventions include vasopressin infusion or catheter-guided embolization.

Emergency surgery is required in 10%–25% of patients with LGIBs, and mortality ranges from 13% to 50%.[10] Indications for surgery include persistent hemodynamic instability with active bleeding or recurrence of active bleeding. Unstable patients may require an emergency exploratory laparotomy with intraoperative endoscopy. In all patients undergoing surgery, an attempt to localize bleeding should be performed (pre- or intraoperatively) because segmental bowel resection is preferred.

Management of Coagulopathies

Vital to the cessation of blood loss is correction of coagulopathy. Anticoagulation medications need to be promptly reversed with the administration of fresh frozen plasma, vitamin K, or prothrombin complex concentrates for warfarin reversal, or protamine sulfate for heparins. Newer oral anticoagulation agents may require hematology assistance for rapid reversal.

In the setting of massive bleeding, platelets and clotting factors are consumed and diluted by the addition of crystalloid and banked blood. Serum platelet levels, prothrombin time (PT)/international normalized ratio (INR), and partial thromboplastic time (PTT) must be ordered on all patients with massive hemorrhage. Patients who require transfusion with 5 or more units of pRBCs should receive empiric fresh frozen plasma and platelet transfusion. Patients with underlying liver disease may have elevated INRs requiring fresh frozen plasma transfusion, and dialysis patients may be administered desmopressin (DDAVP) for underlying platelet dysfunction. Recombinant activated factor VII has been utilized on some occasions for massive hemorrhage, but ideal use is still undefined.

Controversies

Debate exists regarding many therapeutic interventions for patients with UGIB or LGIB, including utilization of a promotility agent (e.g., erythromycin) prior to upper endoscopy, correction of coagulopathy prior to endoscopy, transfusion requirements for hemodynamically stable patients, endoscopic dislodgement of clot with appropriate treatment for the underlying lesion, and second-look endoscopy for all patients. Most specialists agree that promotility agents are not necessary and that correction of coagulopathy should not delay endoscopy. Clot dislodgement to treat the underlying lesion is recommended, and second-look endoscopy is not usually necessary.

Finally, there is also debate regarding permissive hypotension of the patient (accepting SBP80–100 mm Hg) with massive medical hemorrhage. Animal studies show that crystalloid infusions may result in clot dissolution and create a predisposition toward rebleeding. In traumatic hemorrhage, better outcomes with permissive hypotension are noted. It is reasonable to extrapolate these findings to the medical patient with massive bleeding. We recommend resuscitating a patient to either a SBP of at least 90 mmHg or a MAP of 60 mmHg.

Pearls of Care

1. Massive medical hemorrhage is a medical emergency requiring early identification, aggressive resuscitative care, and ultimate control of bleeding mandatory for survival.
2. An elevated Shock Index (HR/SBP > 0.8) may identify patients at risk for decompensation.
3. After crystalloid resuscitation, transfusion of pRBCs should be administered to transient responders (SBP<90mmHg after initial BP increase) or nonresponders (SBP<90mmHg consistently).
4. Rapid reversal of coagulopathies is a potentially life-saving intervention.
5. Surgical evaluation should be performed on all hemodynamically unstable patients with massive hemorrhage.

References

1. American College of Surgeons Committee on Trauma. Shock. In: *Advanced trauma life support for doctors*. 7th ed. First Impression Press; 2004:74.

2. Fallah MA, Prakash C, Edmundowicz S. Acute gastrointestinal bleeding. *Med Clin North Am* 2000;84(5):1183–1208.

3. Vreeberg EM, Snel P, de Bruijne JW, et al. Acute upper gastrointestinal bleeding in the Amsterdam area: incidence, diagnosis and clinical outcome. *Am J Gastroenterol* 1997;92:236–243.

4. Garcia-Tsao G, Bosch J. Current concepts: management of varices and variceal hemorrhage in cirrhosis. *N Engl J Med* 2010;362:823–832.

5. Gayer C, Chino A, Lucas C, et al. Acute lower gastrointestinal bleeding in 1,112 patients admitted to an urban emergency medical center. *Surgery* 2009;146(4):600–606.

6. Vernava AM, Longo WE, Virgo KS. A nationwide study of the incidence and etiology of lower gastrointestinal bleeding. *Surg Res Commun* 1996;18:113–120.

7. Rutledge R, Oller DW, Meyer AA. A statewide, population-based, time series analysis of the outcomes of ruptured aortic aneurysm. *Ann Surg* 1996;223:492–505.

8. Green BT, Rockey DC. Lower gastrointestinal bleeding management. Gastrointest Clin North Am 2005;34:s.

9. Hunter JM, Pezim ME. Limited value of technetium 99m-labeled red cell scintigraphy in localization of lower gastrointestinal bleeding. *Am J Surg* 1990;159(5):504–506.

10. Leitman IM, Paull DE, Shires GT. Evaluation and management of massive lower gastrointestinal hemorrhage. *Ann. Surg* 1989;209(2):175–180.

Selected Readings

Barnert J, Messmann H. Diagnosis and management of lower gastrointestinal bleeding. Nat Rev Gastroenterol Hepatol 2009;6(11):637–646.

Granlnek IM, Barkun AN, Bardou M. Management of acute bleeding from a peptic ulcer. *NEngl J Med* 2008;359:928–937.

Garcia-Tsao G, Bosch J. Current concepts: management of varices and variceal hemorrhage in cirrhosis. *NEngl J Med* 2010;362:823–832.

Lee J, Costantini TW, Coimbra R. Acute lower GI bleeding for the acute care surgeon: current diagnosis and management. *Scand J Surg* 2009;98(3):135–142.

MannuccioMannucci P, Levi M. Prevention and treatment of major bleeding, *NEngl J Med* 2007;356:2301–2311.

Zuckerman GR, Prakash C. Acute lower intestinal bleeding. Part II: etiology, therapy, and outcomes. *Gastrointest Endosc* 1999;49(2):228–238.

Part II

Methodology and Procedures

Chapter 13

Procedural Analgesia and Sedation (Moderate and Deep)

John H. Burton

Introduction

The goal of procedural analgesia is optimizing the performance of the procedure while limiting pain. Often, pain relief alone is sufficient; other procedures may provoke responses that cannot be relieved solely by an analgesic approach alone. In these encounters, a combined analgesic and sedative approach can relieve patient suffering.

Patient sedation for acute procedures can achieve a number of goals in addition to relief of pain and suffering. Muscle relaxation is an important need of many acute procedures, such as reduction of a major joint dislocation. Sedation agents, particularly intravenous sedative medications, can provide muscle relaxation and thus improve both the success of procedures and the pain from active traction against these tissues.

Another frequently encountered factor in the acutely ill or injured patient is anxiety. Quelling anxiety—termed *anxiolysis*—is an essential component to enhancing patient cooperation and optimization of success. A child with an acute facial laceration requiring surgical repair is a common example of a procedure with an anxiolytic need.

Definition of Terms

Procedural analgesia should consider two sources of discomfort: pain that is suffered as a direct consequence of any medical condition, and pain that will be suffered during any procedure. Treating pain with a standard yet tailored approach should be routine. This approach should incorporate analgesics with an emphasis on safety and effectiveness.

Procedural sedation seeks to limit anxiety and to suppress a patient's level of consciousness during a procedure. The intended sedation depth should vary in accordance with the specific needs of the patient and procedure. For example, central line insertion may be done with local anesthesia and light sedation, whereas tube thoracostomy will likely require local anesthesia plus combined systemic analgesia and sedation.

Sedation depths of "mild," "moderate," and "deep" levels of altered consciousness are cited in the medical literature. These descriptors should be visualized as depths along a continuum of sedation. The extreme of this continuum is general anesthesia, whereby unresponsiveness to all stimuli and the absence of airway protective reflexes exist. This is not usually the target of procedural sedation but can occur, even when unintended. Be prepared for this occurrence.

Minimal sedation describes a patient with a near-baseline level of alertness. This level of sedation does not impair the ability to follow commands or respond to verbal stimuli. Under a state of minimal sedation, cardiovascular and ventilatory functions are not threatened or impaired.

Moderate sedation describes a depth of consciousness characterized by many or all of the following: ptosis, slurred speech, and delayed or altered responses to verbal stimuli. Event amnesia is frequent under moderate sedation. The patient's airway and breathing is usually minimally depressed, though vigilance in recognizing deeper depression is required as sedation depth increases. The likelihood of cardiovascular embarrassment is low, but we recommend monitoring of cardiovascular status (oxygenation, blood pressure, and heart rate). Most emergency department (ED) procedures are done with mild or moderate sedation.

Deep sedation renders the patient unresponsive to most verbal commands with an intended preservation of airway protective reflexes and responses to noxious, painful stimuli. Event amnesia is typical of deep levels of sedation. Monitoring for deep sedation encounters should emphasize the potential for reduction in ventilation and cardiovascular complications, including changes to heart rate, heart rhythm, and blood pressure. The potential for respiratory depression and apnea should invoke more sensitive ventilation monitoring techniques, including oxygen saturation and exhaled end-tidal carbon dioxide ($ETCO_2$) levels. Deep sedation is often sought during major joint relocation, cardioversion, or other profoundly noxious events; respiratory depression may be most likely right after completion of a procedure, when nociceptive stimuli are lessened but the drugs remain at peak levels.

Indications

Providers caring for ED patients should have a planned, comprehensive treatment approach. Such an approach should consider preprocedure pain, targeted amount of sedation or anxiolysis, expected pain of the procedure, and patient-specific needs to safely enhance and optimize acute interventions. *Planning must include anticipating complications* (notably respiratory or hemodynamic), and providers should be prepared to recognize and act on these if they occur.

Acute interventions in the ED setting are numerous and a broad categorization of indications for procedural sedation would include the following:

• Orthopedic: acute fracture or dislocation reduction
• Minor general surgery: laceration repair, wound exploration, abscess incision and debridement, wound debridement, foreign body removal, and chest tube thoracostomy

- General medical: central venous line placement, lumbar puncture, electrical cardioversion, radiographic imaging (often computed tomography or magnetic resonance imaging for pediatric patients)

Contraindications

Given the emergent nature of life- and limb-threatening conditions in critically ill patients, *commonly accepted contraindications to moderate and deep levels of patient sedation for elective procedures do not apply well in the ED*. Many illnesses require a rapid intervention to optimize the outcome; this means that risks associated with delays in performing an intervention could outweigh commonly accepted contraindications noted for elective procedures. These contraindications include recent intake of solids or liquids, advanced age, or medical comorbidities.

The consideration of sedative or analgesic agents should incorporate patient-specific risks into both the decision to pursue a specific depth of sedation and the treatment agent selection. Patient screening in preparation for procedural sedation should include the following:

- History of present illness
- Past medical history
- History of allergy or prior anesthetic complications
- Most recent oral intake of liquids and foods
- Physical examination directed toward airway and cardiovascular assessment

Acute or chronic illnesses such as congestive heart failure, history of cerebrovascular accident, valvular heart disease, and seizure may increase the risk for adverse cardiovascular or respiratory events. Obesity, excessive facial hair, or traumatic facial injuries/anatomic limitations may make monitoring or airway rescue difficult if needed. Conditions such as hemorrhagic shock or sepsis may enhance the risk of hypotension.

The timing and need to delay a procedure to "clear" oral intake of fluids or solids prior to sedation (to lessen aspiration risk) is debated in ED procedural analgesia and sedation. The brief periods of suppressed consciousness and lighter depths of sedation during ED procedures limit the applicability of common elective operating-room fasting approaches. The data on ED procedures are limited but delays solely to meet a 4–6 hour fasting threshold are generally not justified for ED procedural analgesia and sedation.

Technique

Patient safety considerations in the treatment of pain should follow a weight-based and titrated analgesic dosing strategy. A weight-based strategy should incorporate the "therapeutic window" for safety and effectiveness, seeking to avoid excessive dosing of medication and subsequent side effects such as respiratory depression while optimizing comfort.

If the painful condition will continue after the procedure, utilize longer acting analgesics such as hydromorphone and morphine. If the pain stimulus will abate or drop dramatically—a common event—a shorter acting analgesic agent such as fentanyl should be considered for procedure-related pain.

An important safety consideration is the awareness that coadministration of analgesics and sedative agents increases the potential for respiratory depression and hemodynamic instability. Simultaneous administration of sedative and analgesic agents is best avoided. *A safer approach is to utilize analgesics first to create an appropriate analgesic endpoint, then titrate sedation as needed* (Fig. 13.1).

Intravenous titration is the preferred method for procedural analgesia and sedation. Ketamine is one agent for which this may be an exception, with data supporting intravenous or intramuscular use. Intravenous dosing is typically done as bolus followed by subsequent repeat bolus-dosing of smaller increments (one-third to one-half the initial dose) titrated to the desired clinical effect.

Selection and Dosing of Sedation Agent

Sedative agents utilized for light sedation include the following drugs and initial intravenous dosing strategies (followed by titration as needed):

- Fentanyl (confers analgesia and sedation): 2–4 mcg/kg
- Midazolam: 0.03 mg/kg
- Lorazepam: 0.02 mg/kg

Sedative agents utilized for moderate levels of sedation include the following drugs and initial intravenous dosing strategies:

- Midazolam: 0.05 mg/kg
- Ketamine: 0.5 mg/kg (2–4 mg/kg if intramuscular used)

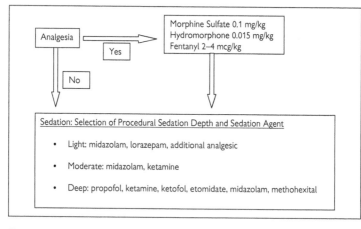

Figure 13.1 Weight-based dosing approach for analgesia administration prior to sedation agent selection and administration.

Deep sedation utilizes agents and dosing that can progress into depths of altered consciousness associated with general anesthesia. Sedative agents utilized for deep levels of sedation include the following drugs and initial intravenous dosing strategies:

- Midazolam: 0.075 mg/kg
- Ketamine: 1.0 mg/kg
- Propofol: 1.0 mg/kg
- Ketamine/propofol combination: intravenous, 0.5 mg/kg, respectively
- Etomidate: 0.15 mg/kg
- Methohexital: 1.0 mg/kg

Coadministration of midazolam and fentanyl is frequently utilized to induce moderate or deep levels of sedation. Many recent studies demonstrated increased adverse outcomes, particularly respiratory depression and apnea, with this combination. Newer approaches deploying short-acting sedation agents such as propofol, ketamine, or etomidate with an analgesic allow safer and shorter procedural sedation.

"Ketofol" is the moniker for a combination of ketamine and propofol administered as a single bolus after mixing 1:1 (mg and mg, respectively) in the same syringe. Dosing of the combination is less than the use of propofol or ketamine alone, approximately 0.5–0.75 mg/kg for each agent. The advantage of this combination strategy is less hypotension and respiratory depression. Ketamine alone is emetogenic, but in combination with low-dose propofol this effect is offset.

Monitoring Sedation Depth

Monitoring sedation depth is best done by serial exam along with monitoring equipment. The exam should be structured, using a standardized sedation assessment scale. The Modified Sedation Agitation Score and the Ramsay Scale are patient sedation scales commonly utilized for sedation assessment (Fig. 13.2). A sedation assessment instrument should utilize a validated set of patient assessment markers. These markers should be age-relevant given the wide disparity in application for patient evaluation across patient populations.

Avoiding Complications

The immediate availability of ventilation and cardiovascular monitoring and support equipment is essential as the likelihood of complications increases with deeper levels of unconsciousness. A defibrillator, continuous suction, bag-valve mask, nasal and oral airway adjuncts, and intubation equipment should be at the bedside and prepared for immediate use when complications are encountered.

The need for a dedicated practitioner, separate from the provider(s) performing the procedure, who has the ability to recognize and intervene with airway or hemodynamic changes is mandatory, especially when using anything beyond light sedation. Given the potential for many sedation agents to invoke

Ramsay Score	
Score	**Description**
1	Patient anxious, agitated, or restless
2	Patient cooperative, oriented, and tranquil
3	Patient responding only to verbal commands
4	Patient with brisk response to light glabella tap or loud auditory stimulus
5	Patient with sluggish response to light glabella tap or loud auditory stimulus
6	Patient with no response to light glabella tap or loud auditory stimulus

Sedation-Agitation Score		
Score	**Description**	**Response**
7	Dangerous agitation	Pulling at endotracheal tube, thrashing, climbing over bed rails
6	Very agitated	Does not calm, requires restraints, bites endotracheal tube
5	Agitated	Attempts to sit up but calms to verbal instructions
4	Calm and cooperative	Obeys commands
3	Sedated	Difficult to rouse, obeyss simple commands
2	Very sedated	Rouses to stimuli. Does not obey commands
1	Unarousable	Minimal or no response to noxious stimuli

Figure 13.2 Modified Sedation-Agitation Scale and Ramsay Score for the assessment of sedation level. (Riker 1999; Ramsay 1974)

deep sedation levels and general anesthesia, the use of a dedicated sedation provider for all moderate and deep sedation is encouraged.

General and Key Management Controversies

Deep Sedation Providers

Given the acknowledgment that short-acting, powerful sedative drugs such as propofol can induce general anesthesia even when the target depth is moderate or deep, attention to the qualifications and settings appropriate for the use of deep sedation-provoking drugs are important. Current research supports that trained emergency physicians in an appropriate setting and with the right tools provide effective and safe deep sedation. However, large registries to deliver more granular insights and risks—like those available in the operating room literature—do not yet exist. A pragmatic and safe approach would be that deep sedation practices should involve medical professionals with training that include rescue expertise for both airway and cardiovascular compromise coupled with close quality assurance and reporting.

Routine Use of Capnography

The routine use of capnography for $ETCO_2$ monitoring has been a subject of great debate in the medical literature for procedural sedation. Adoption of this technology for routine use will incur expense for devices and personnel training with uncertain patient safety advantages.

Advocates for routine $ETCO_2$ monitoring cite the enhanced sensitivity of this technology for the detection of respiratory depression and apnea. Capnography represents a continuous assessment of ventilation and can detect apnea that is missed by clinical observation alone during procedural sedation encounters. Opponents cite the lack of specificity of these brief apnea events with uncertain clinical relevance for many of the detected events. Currently, most agree that capnography should be used in all deep sedation cases, and it may be withheld or used in selected cases for light or moderate sedation.

Recent Oral Ingestion

The emergent or critical nature of many procedures in the emergency environment has provoked debate over the relevance of commonly utilized anesthesia oral intake policies (NPO policies) when applied to procedural sedation outside of the operating room setting.

Vomiting and aspiration risks are proportional to the depth of sedation. However, data in the ED procedural sedation literature do not link a high frequency of aspiration or poor outcomes related to aspiration with nonadherence to traditional NPO policies. Opponents believe that this finding represents underreporting of events.

The emergent nature of many ED procedures demands a risk/benefit balance that must be considered with recent oral intake policies. The application of a minimum 4–6 hour delay for patients undergoing emergent procedures may alter outcomes negatively without adding meaningful safety. No one rule will suffice always; it is best that the risks of procedure delay be weighed against the aspiration risk in each specific patient encounter, particularly those involving deep sedation levels.

Pearls of Care

1. Procedural systemic analgesia and sedation must be planned, with a clearly targeted depth based, on the anticipated adverse effects.
2. The simultaneous administration of analgesics and sedative agents increases the potential for adverse events, particularly respiratory depression, respiratory arrest, and hemodynamic instability. Titrate analgesia first, then assess the need for sedation and target that outcome.
3. Deep sedation encounters should be performed in a highly monitored environment with a provider trained in rescue airway and hemodynamic interventions and with nearby resuscitative equipment.

Table 13.1 Common Moderate and Deep Procedural Sedation Agents, Dosing, and Considerations for Each Agent

Agent	Initial Dose (mg/kg)	Repeat Dose (mg/kg)	Consideration(s)
Midazolam	0.05	0.03	Titrate to desired depth; patient response is variable
Etomidate	0.15	0.1	Myoclonus may render inappropriate for cardioversion and imaging procedures
Propofol	0.5–1.0	0.5	Caution for use in patients with hemodynamic instability due to reduction in central venous pressure
Ketamine/propofol "Ketafol"	0.5/0.5	0.25/0.25	Agents should be combined in same syringe for simultaneous administration
Ketamine	1.0	0.5	Vomiting may be reduced with coadministration of ondansetron; emergence reactions may render inappropriate for adults

4. Administration of agents for analgesia and sedation should follow a weight-based and titrated medication dosing strategy, with simultaneous consideration of patient age and comorbidities. Titration is best performed using an intravenous bolus followed by repeat bolus-dosing of smaller increments until reaching the desired sedation level.

5. Watch for respiratory depression immediately after a painful procedure is completed—this is when drug effect is high but stimuli low.

Selected Readings

American Society of Anesthesiologists, Task Force on Sedation and Analgesia by Non-Anesthesiologists. Practice guidelines for sedation and analgesia by non-anesthesiologists. Anesthes 2002;96:1004–1017.

Burton JH, Harrah JD, Germann CA, Dillon DC. Does end-tidal carbon dioxide monitoring detect respiratory events prior to current sedation monitoring practices? Acad Emerg Med 2006;13:500–504.

Burton JH, Miner JR, Shipley ER, Strout TD, Becker C, Thode HC. Propofol for emergency department procedural sedation and analgesia: a tale of three centers. Acad Emerg Med 2006;13:24–30.

Chung F. Discharge criteria—a new trend. Can J Anaesth 1995;11:1056–1058.

Deitch KR, Chudnofsky CR, Dominici P. The utility of supplemental oxygen during emergency department procedural sedation with Propofol: a randomized, controlled trial. Ann Emerg Med 2007;49:1–8.

Green SM, Roback MG, Miner JR, Burton JH, Krauss B. Fasting and emergency department procedural sedation and analgesia: a consensus-based clinical practice advisory. Ann Emerg Med 2007;49:454–461.

Miner JR, Burton JH. Clinical practice advisory: emergency department procedural sedation with Propofol. *Ann Emerg Med* 2007;50:182–187.

Miner JR, Gray RO, Bahr J, Patel R, McGill JW. Randomized clinical trial of Propofol versus ketamine for procedural sedation in the emergency department. *Acad Emerg Med* 2010;17:604–611.

Miner JR, Martel ML, Meyer M, Reardon R, Biros MH. Procedural sedation of critically ill patients in the emergency department. *Acad Emerg Med* 2005;12:124–128.

Phillips W, Anderson A, Rosengreen M, Johnson J, Halpin J. Propofol versus Propofol/ketamine for brief painful procedures in the emergency department: clinical and bispectral index scale comparison. *J Pain Palliat Care Pharmacother* 2010;24:349–355.

Ramsay MAE, Savege TM, Simpson BRJ, and Goodwin R. Controlled sedation with alphaxalone-alphadolone. *Br Med J.* 1974; 2: 656–659.

Riker RR, Picard JT, Fraser GL. Prospective evaluation of the sedation-agitation scale for adult critically ill patients. *Crit Care Med* 1999;27:1325–1329

Chapter 14

Monitoring Technology
Invasive and Noninvasive

H. Bryant Nguyen

Indications

The purpose of hemodynamic monitoring is to identify and guide therapy in the unstable patient. Therapy includes resuscitation, afterload optimization, and if needed, inotropic support. Vital signs, including heart rate and arterial blood pressure, do not assess the adequacy of tissue perfusion. Delaying shock resuscitation until a patient develops hypotension is too late because tissue ischemia has already occurred. Therefore, hemodynamic variables beyond traditional vital signs allow the clinician to differentiate various causes of hemodynamic instability and to intervene appropriately. Advanced monitoring techniques can serve as diagnostic aids and can provide therapeutic targets for patient management.

Pulmonary artery catheterization has been the reference standard for hemodynamic monitoring since the early 1970s. However, its invasiveness and lack of outcome benefit have made the pulmonary artery catheter (PAC) less common in the management of critically ill patients. Also, PAC is somewhat impractical to impliment in the emergency setting. On the other hand, the need to know central hemodynamics, including cardiac output (CO), can be crucial during resuscitation. In the emergency department (ED) setting, the study of early goal-directed therapy in septic shock has advanced hemodynamic monitoring utilizing central venous pressure (CVP), mean arterial pressure (MAP), and central venous oxygen saturation (ScvO$_2$) in patients with hypotension refractory to initial fluid resuscitation or with significant lactic acidosis.[1] While this approach has been best studied in septic shock, the physiologic rationale for hemodynamic monitoring would apply to any patient with persistent hypotension and/or significant organ hypoperfusion. Table 14.1 illustrates the various hemodynamic variables currently obtainable in the ED.

In resuscitation of the shock patient, a few practical rules are worth keeping in mind[2]:

- Tachycardia is never a good thing.
- Hypotension is always pathologic.
- Central venous pressure is only elevated in disease.

Table 14.1 Hemodynamic Variables Obtainable in the Emergency Department

Hemodynamic Variable	Method of Measurement
Hemoglobin oxygen saturation, %	Pulse oximetry, arterial blood gas
Heart rate, beats/min	Physical examination, pulse oximetry, electrocardiography
Blood pressure, mm Hg	Sphygmomanometry, oscillometry, intra-arterial catherization
Central venous pressure (CVP), mm Hg	Jugular venous pulsation, ultrasound, central venous catherization
Cardiac output (CO), L/min	Thoracic bioimpedance or bioreactance, transesophageal or transcutaneous Doppler ultrasound, transesophageal or transthoracic echocardiography, pulse contour analysis, lithium dilution, transpulmonary (arterial) thermodilution, pulmonary artery thermodilution
Central venous oxygen saturation (ScvO$_2$), %	Central venous catherization for intermittent venous blood sampling or continuous measurement
Lactate, mmol/L	Arterial, venous, or capillary sampling

- There is no such thing as a normal cardiac output.
- Peripheral edema is only of cosmetic concern.

Most important, however, no hemodynamic monitoring technology in itself will improve outcome unless clinicians use that data to identify the underlying disease process and initiate effective therapies for that particular disease process.

Contraindications

The current state of the art in hemodynamic monitoring includes invasive techniques of central venous or arterial catheter insertion using the Seldinger approach. Absolute contraindications to either arterial or venous catheter insertion include the following:

- Infection, such as cellulitis at the insertion site
- Ischemia or arterial insufficiency local to the insertion site
- Trauma adjacent to the insertion site, such as an extremity fracture
- Artificial graft at the insertion site
- Evidence of anatomic obstruction, including thrombosis of the same extremity, superior vena cava syndrome on the side of an upper chest catheter insertion site, and tumor in close proximity to the insertion site

Relative contraindications to consider prior to placing an arterial or venous catheter include the following:

- Coagulopathy, with international normalized ratio >1.5
- Thrombocytopenia, with platelet count <50,000/µL

- Another existing catheter, including pacemaker and internal defibrillator wires, on the same side as an upper chest catheter
- High level of positive end-expiratory pressure in a mechanically ventilated patient when inserting a subclavian catheter
- Tracheostomy and/or excessive secretions when inserting an internal jugular vein catheter

Several noninvasive technologies are available for hemodynamic monitoring. These technologies often involve skin electrodes, sensors, or probes to obtain hemodynamic measurements. The contraindication to using these devices would generally include any possible allergic reaction to the materials being applied on the skin. Patient comfort is a final consideration prior to using any hemodynamic monitoring technology, invasive or noninvasive.

Techniques

Arterial Blood Pressure Monitoring

The circulatory analogy of Ohm's Law states that the arterial pressure is proportional to CO (or blood flow in liters per minute) and total peripheral resistance (TPR):

- Mean arterial pressure (MAP) = CO x TPR.
- MAP can be estimated as the sum of the diastolic pressure and one-third of the pulse pressure.
- Systolic pressure is the maximum pressure during ventricular ejection.
- Diastolic pressure is the lowest pressure in the blood vessels during ventricular filling.

Blood pressure may be normal in the presence of low cardiac output with preserved vasomotor tone. However, hypotension is always pathological and reflects a failure of normal circulatory compensatory mechanisms.

Noninvasive Measurement

Palpation of an arterial pulse in an emergency situation can provide an estimated minimum systolic pressure:

- Radial pulse approximates 80 mm Hg
- Femoral pulse approximates 70 mm Hg
- Carotid pulse approximates 60 mm Hg

Auscultation for blood pressure began with the invention of the sphygmomanometer by Scipione Riva-Rocci in 1896. Appropriate cuff size, cuff placement, placement of the stethoscope bell, cuff deflation rate, auscultation of Korotkoff sounds, dysrhythmia, observer bias, and faulty equipment all contribute to variability in the auscultatory method. In choosing a cuff size, the following points need to be considered:

- The cuff width should be 40% of the upper arm circumference.
- The cuff bladder length should be 80% of the upper arm circumference.

- A small cuff for the size of the arm results in falsely elevated blood pressure.
- A large cuff for the size of the arm results in falsely low blood pressure.

   The oscillometric method is provided by most patient monitors used in the ED setting. The amplitude of the fluctuations (or oscillations) in blood pressure in a sphygmomanometer cuff is analyzed and converted to pressure measurements by a computer device without the need for auscultation with the stethoscope. Controversy exists regarding the accuracy of oscillometric blood pressure monitors. When in doubt, manual sphygmomanometric measurement of blood pressure is recommended.

Invasive Measurement

Noninvasive blood pressure measurements can underestimate systolic pressure by more than 30 mm Hg in the hypotensive vasoconstricted patient. Thus, intra-arterial blood pressure monitoring provides more accurate assessment of cardiovascular instability during resuscitation, especially in patients with refractory shock receiving vasoactive agents. Common sites for arterial catheterization include the radial artery and femoral artery. Other sites include axillary, brachial, dorsalis pedis, ulnar, tibial posterialis, and temporal arteries. While using the Allen test to confirm collateral blood flow prior to radial artery catheterization is recommended, it does not predict who will develop ischemic complications well. Peripheral vascular disease, shock, and vasoactive drug use increase risk of distal ischemia.

   After successful arterial catheterization, connection of the catheter to the pressure transducer should reveal an arterial waveform. The square-wave flush test is applied to determine whether artifacts in the tubing and recording system are damping the pressure measurements (Fig. 14.1). Further flushing of the system or tubing replacement may be required to remove air bubbles.

   During resuscitation of shock, the optimal MAP varies depending on the underlying cause of hemodynamic instability. The International Consensus Conference recommended these as targets[3]:

- MAP of 40 mm Hg in uncontrolled hemorrhage due to trauma
- MAP of 90 mm Hg for traumatic brain injury
- MAP greater than 65 mm Hg for other forms of shock

Central Venous Pressure Monitoring

CVP is the resistance to systemic venous return, with high values indicating larger than normal volume returning to the heart from the systemic circulation. Clinically, it is an indicator of central blood volume and right atrial pressure. A multitude of studies, commentaries, and editorials have been written debating the validity of a CVP target in critically ill patients. Most clinicians accept that a low CVP indicates hypovolemia, whereas an elevated measurement suggests volume overload. Others will argue that a single CVP measurement is useless and factors such as cardiac output, intrathoracic pressure, vascular compliance,

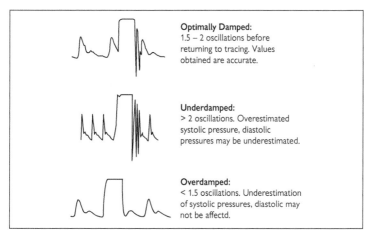

Figure 14.1 Square-wave flush test with intra-arterial blood pressure measurement. During a flush bolus of the catheter tubing, a square wave is observed. The number of oscillations following the square wave at the end of the bolus and prior to returning of the blood pressure tracing may result in an overestimated or underestimated blood pressure.

Reprinted with permission from John Frazier, Edwards Lifesciences, Irvine, Calif: McGee WT et al. *Quick guide to cardiopulmonary care.* Edwards Lifesciences 2009; p. 36.

waveform analysis, dysrhythmia, tricuspid regurgitation or stenosis, and proper transducer placement all contribute to its measurement.

Invasive Measurement

CVP is monitored with a catheter inserted in the internal jugular or subclavian vein proximal to the right atrium with the distal tip in the superior vena cava. Other indications for central venous catheterization include the following:

- Fluid and vasopressor administration
- Frequent blood draws
- Unsuccessful or inadequate peripheral venous access
- Central venous oxygenation ($ScvO_2$) measurement
- Pulmonary artery catheterization
- Transvenous pacemaker placement

After successful catheter insertion using the Seldinger technique and radiographic verification, a continuous CVP waveform is displayed on the bedside monitor with the catheter connected to a pressure transducer. The transducer should be placed at the level of the right atrium, or approximately 5 cm below the sternal angle. The measurement should be taken at the end of expiration. At this point in the respiratory cycle, whether spontaneous or with positive pressure mechanical ventilation, intrapleural pressure is minimal and CVP closely approximates cardiac

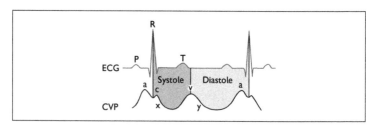

Figure 14.2 Central venous pressure (CVP) waveform and its relationship to the electro-cardiogram (ECG). The *c-wave* represents bulging of the tricuspid valve into the right atrium and occurs at the onset of systole. The base of the *c-wave* is used to determine a CVP value because it is the final pressure in the ventricle before the onset of contraction, reflecting *preload*. The measurement should be taken at end of expiration.

transmural pressure. Recognizing an acceptable CVP waveform will allow the clinician to accurately interpret the measured values (Fig. 14.2).

Measurement of CVP from the internal jugular or subclavian vein is the ideal method. However, at times the less preferred method of femoral vein catheterization is used to measure CVP, such as in patients with coagulopathy or in patients in whom subclavian and/or internal jugular vein catheterization was unsuccessful or resulted in a complication. While CVP measurement via the femoral vein is discouraged, studies suggest that femoral vein pressures do approximate CVP. Similarly, changes in venous pressure measured from a large peripheral vein with few valves may correlate with changes in CVP.

Noninvasive Measurement

The physical exam finding of internal jugular venous pulsation remains an acceptable method to estimate right atrial pressure or CVP. The sternal angle is roughly 5 cm above the center of the right atrium regardless of the patient's position. With the patient sitting at a 45° angle, 5 cm (distance from the sternal angle to the right atrium) is added to the vertical distance between the jugular pulsation and the sternal angle to estimate CVP in cm H_2O.

Ultrasound can be used to provide a noninvasive estimate of CVP in the ED. The right internal jugular vein is viewed with a high-frequency linear transducer (7 to 9 MHz). The longitudinal plane of the vein is examined. The jugular venous pulse is the site where the vein tapers, resembling the neck of a wine bottle. The vertical distance in centimeters between this point of vein collapse and the sternal angle is measured and added to 5 cm to obtain a CVP measurement in cm H_2O.[4]

Cardiac Output Monitoring

Oxygen delivery is a direct function of arterial oxygen content and CO. Perfusion pressure is the most important driving force determining CO in the circulation.

Since the primary goal of resuscitation from shock is to reverse tissue hypoperfusion, CO is often considered the ideal hemodynamic target to improve organ perfusion and oxygen delivery.

Invasive Measurement

Cardiac output is traditionally measured invasively with pulmonary artery catheterization using the thermodilution method. Complications from pulmonary artery catheter (PAC) insertion are similar to those of central venous catheterization. Additional complications include the following:

- Cardiac perforation
- Pulmonary artery perforation
- Tricuspid and pulmonary valve injury
- Knotting of the catheter
- Dysrhythmia and heart block

The clinical utility and outcome benefit of PA catheterization in intensive care patients has been debated for many years since Connors et al. observed that its application was possibly associated with increased mortality and utilization of resources.[5] The benefit of the PAC as a hemodynamic monitoring tool in the ED setting has not been investigated. A less invasive method of measuring cardiac output is perhaps more attractive and practical.

Noninvasive Measurement

Noninvasive techniques to measure CO are an alternative to invasive measurements with the PAC. Table 14.1 illustrates the various methods of measuring CO. Some techniques are minimally invasive, such as intra-arterial pulse pressure waveform analysis to measure cardiac output. Other techniques are truly noninvasive, such as thoracic electrical bioimpedance using skin electrodes to obtain cardiac output based on electrical impedance (or resistance) measured across the chest wall. Multiple studies have examined the reliability, accuracy, and utility of these techniques. However, no technique has been successfully incorporated into a treatment protocol affecting outcome in critically ill patients presenting to the ED.

Determining Fluid Responsiveness

Fluid responsiveness can guide the clinical decision to administer more fluids or, instead, to initiate vasoactive therapy to optimize CO, blood pressure, and organ perfusion. An increase in CO of greater than 15% after a fluid challenge has been considered the gold standard reflecting fluid responsiveness. According to Starling's Law (Fig. 14.3), when CO does not increase in response to fluid therapy, cardiac contractility has reached a plateau and further fluid resuscitation can result in volume overload and pulmonary edema. There is no single optimal CO value, and resuscitation is guided by the relative change in CO in response to therapy.

Changes in CVP can be used to estimate a patient's volume status using the classical description of the "5–2 rule" by Weil et al.[6–7]:

- A 10 to 20 mL/min bolus of normal saline is infused for 10 to 15 minutes (e.g., 250 mL over 15 minutes).
- An increase in CVP >5 mm Hg indicates volume overload and discontinuation of fluid.
- An increase in CVP of 2 to 5 mm Hg indicates fluid should be held and the CVP reevaluated after 10 minutes.
- An increase in CVP <2 mm Hg indicates hypovolemia and a second fluid challenge is justified.

Consider the effects of the respiratory cycle when examining a continuous CVP measurement. Significant variation in CVP measurements between inspiration and expiration suggest that the heart walls are still compliant and will most likely respond to volume infusion. When there is no respiratory variation in CVP, the heart is on the flat part of the cardiac function curve and will no longer respond to fluids.[8]

Sitting up and passive leg raising (PLR) are hydrostatic challenges that can further address volume responsiveness in spontaneously breathing patients and in those with dysrhythmias. Both transiently increase venous return to the heart. The legs are raised to 30 degrees above the chest and held for 1 minute. This maneuver approximates a 200 to 300 mL blood bolus in a 70 kg patient that persists for approximately 2 to 3 minutes. Changes in heart rate, blood pressure, CVP, or cardiac output after PLR are sensitive and specific in predicting volume responsiveness.[9]

Central Venous Oxygen Saturation

Optimal blood pressure and cardiac output are not the only determinants of optimal oxygen delivery and organ perfusion. Mixed-venous oxygen saturation monitoring is a method to assess tissue oxygen extraction and the balance between oxygen delivery (DO_2) and oxygen consumption (VO_2). A normal oxygen extraction ratio (OER) of 25%–35% results in a *venous* oxygen content (reflected in venous oxygen saturation) of approximately 70% of arterial DO_2. Venous oxygen saturation is ideally measured in the pulmonary artery as a mixed venous sample (SvO_2). Clinically, low SvO_2 values reflect inadequate DO_2 and/or excessive VO_2.

Central venous oxygen saturation ($ScvO_2$) measured via a central venous catheter in the jugular or subclavian vein is an alternative to SvO_2. $ScvO_2$ can be easily measured by drawing a standard venous blood gas from the distal port of the central line and obtaining a *measured* oxygen saturation. Continuous measurement can be performed using specialized catheters and monitors equipped with infrared oximetry and reflection spectrophotometry. These catheters provide combined CVP and $ScvO_2$ monitoring.

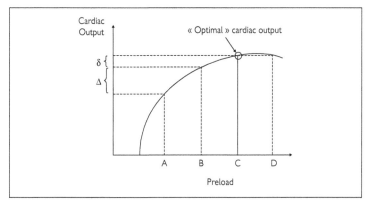

Figure 14.3 Starling's cardiac function curve illustrating the effects of increased preload on cardiac output. The first increase in preload (from A to B) results in a large increase in cardiac output (Δ) as the cardiovascular system operates in the "preload-dependent" portion of the curve. The second increase in preload (from B to C) only results in a small increase in cardiac output (δ), and further increase in preload (from C to D) does not yield any increase in cardiac output as the cardiovascular system is now considered "volume resuscitated" or preload independent.

Reprinted with permission from Wiley-Blackwell Publishing: Cholley BP, Singer M. Esophageal Doppler: noninvasive cardiac output monitor. *Echocardiography* 2003;20:763–769.

When compared to SvO_2, $ScvO_2$ only reflects the oxygen balance for the upper portion of the body and does not include venous return from the coronary sinus. In shock states, $ScvO_2$ is typically 5%–10% *higher* than SvO_2 as blood flow is redistributed from the abdominal vascular beds to the cerebral and coronary circulation. Although absolute values of $ScvO_2$ and SvO_2 may be different, low values of either measurement reflect an imbalance in oxygen transport and portend worse outcomes. Most important, the two measures typically change in parallel and *trends* in $ScvO_2$ reflect trends in SvO_2.[10]

The principal value of $ScvO_2$ is its ability to detect occult inadequate DO_2 relative to VO_2, regardless of the underlying pathophysiologic state (e.g., heart failure, septic shock, trauma). Despite normalization of vital signs and urine output, low $ScvO_2$ can reflect global tissue hypoxia. However, normal or high $ScvO_2$, on the other hand, does not guarantee adequate perfusion because regional areas of tissue hypoperfusion still can be present. Additionally, in several disease states (e.g., hypothermia, terminal shock, cyanide poisoning), shunt conditions, or with cellular metabolic dysfunction, a high $ScvO_2$ can exist despite profound shock.[11]

Lactate

In critical illness, when DO_2 is inadequate to meet tissue oxygen demand and compensatory mechanisms are exhausted, anaerobic metabolism produces lactate. Numerous studies since 1960s have established the use of lactate as a prognostic marker in the critically ill patients with various forms of shock.[12]

When interpreting an elevated lactate level in a patient presenting to the ED, etiologies other than shock and tissue hypoxia must be considered[13]:

- Seizure
- Diabetic ketoacidosis
- Malignancy
- Thiamine deficiency
- Malaria
- HIV infection
- Carbon monoxide
- Cyanide poisoning
- Mitochondrial myopathies
- Metformin
- Simvastatin
- Lactulose
- Antiretroviral
- Niacin
- Isoniazid
- Linezolid

Blood lactate concentrations reflect the interaction between its production and elimination. A critically ill patient with hepatic dysfunction may have a higher lactate level compared with another patient without liver disease, due to impaired hepatic clearance. However, without an acute insult these patients do not commonly have a high lactate level.[14] Thus, lactate elevation in a patient with chronic liver disease suggests the presence of shock and still portends poor prognosis.

A lactate level greater than or equal to 4 mmol/L in a seemingly stable normotensive is associated with increased intensive care unit admission rates and mortality.[15] Furthermore, persistent elevations in lactate lasting more than 24 hours are associated with increased mortality as high as 90%.[16] As an organ perfusion target in the ED setting, the ability to decrease lactate (or lactate clearance) as early as 6 hours in patients with severe sepsis or septic shock is associated with increased 60-day survival.[17,18]

Complications

Any invasive procedure performed in the acute setting of the ED has inherent complications that the clinician must be aware of. Table 14.2 and Table 14.3 illustrate the potential complications associated with arterial and venous catheterization.[19–21]

Understanding the anatomic landmarks, proper preparation and insertion techniques are required to avoid complications. Ultrasound guidance for internal

Table 14.2 Complications of Intra-Arterial Catheterization

	Radial Artery	Femoral Artery	Axillary Artery
Permanent ischemia	0.1	0.2	0.2
Temporary occlusion	19.7	1.5	1.2
Sepsis	0.1	0.4	0.5
Local infection	0.7	0.8	2.2
Pseudoaneurysm	0.1	0.3	0.1
Hematoma	14.4	6.1	2.3
Bleeding	0.5	1.6	1.4

Data are presented as percent.

jugular vein catheter insertion may reduce the number of punctures, improve patient comfort, and decrease the risk for complications.[22] Implementing a central line *bundle* has been advocated to prevent catheter-related infection[23]:

• Hand washing with soap or an alcohol-based sanitizer
• Full barrier precautions during the insertion, including cap, mask, sterile gown, and sterile gloves, for the operator and assistant
• Cleaning the skin with chlorhexidine, and not betadine
• Avoiding the femoral site

Pearls of Care

1. Use multiple data points to assess shock presence or response to therapy-blood pressure, CVP, ScvO2, lactate – all linked to the patients condition. Any one can fail to detect profound illness.

Table 14.3 Complications of Central Venous Catheterization

	Internal Jugular Vein	Subclavian Vein	Femoral Vein
Arterial puncture	6.3–9.4	3.–4.9	9.0–15.0
Hematoma	<0.1–2.2	1.2–2.1	3.8–4.4
Hemothorax	N/A	0.4–0.6	N/A
Pneumothorax	<0.1–0.2	1.5–3.1	N/A
Local infection	4.6	1.4	13.2
Blood stream infection	1.8	0.9	6.9

Data are presented as percent.

2. CVP is best used to assess responsiveness to therapy unless markedly elevated (>16 mmHg.).
3. Target mean arterial pressure of >65 mmHg, not a simple systolic blood pressure, during shock care.

References

1. Rivers E, Nguyen B, Havstad S, et al. Early goal-directed therapy in the treatment of severe sepsis and septic shock. *N Engl J Med* 2001;345:1368–1377.

2. Pinsky MR. Hemodynamic evaluation and monitoring in the ICU. *Chest* 2007;132:2020–2029.

3. Antonelli M, Levy M, Andrews PJ, et al. Hemodynamic monitoring in shock and implications for management. International Consensus Conference, Paris, France, 27–28 April 2006. Intensive Care Med 2007;33:575–590.

4. Lipton B. Estimation of central venous pressure by ultrasound of the internal jugular vein. *Am J Emerg Med* 2000;18:432–434.

5. Connors AF, Jr., Speroff T, Dawson NV, et al. The effectiveness of right heart catheterization in the initial care of critically ill patients. SUPPORT Investigators. *JAMA* 1996;276:889–897.

6. Weil MH, Shubin H, Rosoff L. Fluid repletion in circulatory shock: central venous pressure and other practical guides. *JAMA* 1965;192:668–674.

7. Vincent JL, Weil MH. Fluid challenge revisited. *Crit Care Med* 2006;34:1333–1337.

8. Westphal GA, Silva E, Caldeira Filho M, Roman Goncalves AR, Poli-de-Figueiredo LF. Variation in amplitude of central venous pressure curve induced by respiration is a useful tool to reveal fluid responsiveness in postcardiac surgery patients. *Shock* 2006;26:140–145.

9. Monnet X, Rienzo M, Osman D, et al. Passive leg raising predicts fluid responsiveness in the critically ill. *Crit Care Med* 2006;34:1402–1407.

10. Marx G, Reinhart K. Venous oximetry. *Curr Opin Crit Care* 2006;12:263–268.

11. Rivers EP, Ander DS, Powell D. Central venous oxygen saturation monitoring in the critically ill patient. *Curr Opin Crit Care* 2001;7:204–211.

12. Huckabee WE. Abnormal resting blood lactate, I. The significance of hyperlactemia in hospitalized patients. *Am J Med* 1961;30:833.

13. Fall PJ, Szerlip HM. Lactic acidosis: from sour milk to septic shock. *J Intensive Care Med* 2005;20:255–271.

14. Kruse JA, Zaidi SA, Carlson RW. Significance of blood lactate levels in critically ill patients with liver disease. *Am J Med* 1987;83:77–82.

15. Aduen J, Bernstein WK, Khastgir T, et al. The use and clinical importance of a substrate-specific electrode for rapid determination of blood lactate concentrations. *JAMA* 1994;272:1678–1685.

16. Bakker J, Gris P, Coffernils M, Kahn RJ, Vincent JL. Serial blood lactate levels can predict the development of multiple organ failure following septic shock. *Am J Surg* 1996;171:221–226.

17. Nguyen HB, Rivers EP, Knoblich BP, et al. Early lactate clearance is associated with improved outcome in severe sepsis and septic shock. *Crit Care Med* 2004;32:1637–1642.

18. Arnold RC, Shapiro NI, Jones AE, et al. Multi-center study of early lactate clearance as a determinant of survival in patients with presumed sepsis. *Shock* 2009;32:35–39.

19. Scheer B, Perel A, Pfeiffer UJ. Clinical review: complications and risk factors of peripheral arterial catheters used for haemodynamic monitoring in anaesthesia and intensive care medicine. *Crit Care* 2002;6:199–204.

20. McGee DC, Gould MK. Preventing complications of central venous catheterization. *N Engl J Med* 2003;348:1123–1133.

21. Lorente L, Henry C, Martin MM, Jimenez A, Mora ML. Central venous catheter-related infection in a prospective and observational study of 2,595 catheters. *Crit Care* 2005;9:R631–R635.

22. Balls A, LoVecchio F, Kroeger A, Stapczynski JS, Mulrow M, Drachman D. Ultrasound guidance for central venous catheter placement: results from the Central Line Emergency Access Registry Database. *Am J Emerg Med* 2010;28:561–567.

23. Pronovost P, Needham D, Berenholtz S, et al. An intervention to decrease catheter-related bloodstream infections in the ICU. *N Engl J Med* 2006;355:2725–2732.

Chapter 15

Airway Management

Henry E. Wang and Jestin N. Carlson

Introduction

Airway management is a fundamental step in the management of the critically ill. While endotracheal intubation (ETI) is the standard modality for the critically ill, the emergency physician must be familiar with a range of alternative airway management strategies and techniques.

General Considerations

Characteristics of a Potentially Difficult Intubation

These factors may indicate patients who will offer airway management challenges:

- Obesity
- Short neck
- Small mouth
- Over/underbite
- Limited neck mobility
- Airway trauma or injury
- Anatomical anomalies
  These clinical situations may increase the difficulty of airway management:
- Head or other major injury
- Hypotension
- Intoxicated or combative patient
- Anaphylaxis
- Stridor
- Angioedema or any swelling

Airway difficulty should be anticipated and identified early. *Plan for failure* and do not persist in any one failing approach when the aforementioned factors exist.

Airway Management Planning and Decision Making

Airway management is a complex time-critical process involving multiple steps. Accumulated delays can result in loss of airway control and harm. It is imperative that care teams plan all steps of airway management in advance, before the initiation of interventions. The bedside provider should adhere to a few guiding principles:

- *Assess the patient early*—before the onset of airway crisis.
- *Prepare early*—before the actual need for interventions.
- *Anticipate airway difficulty.* Some believe that all emergent airways should be considered "difficult" airways.
- *Establish clear airway management plans,* including the planned sequence of laryngoscopy techniques and rescue airway interventions prior to the first intubation attempt. Rescue supraglottic airways or surgical airway equipment should be immediately available at the bedside.
- *Change intubation equipment, technique, or operator* with each intubation attempt—avoid repeating the same unsuccessful approach.
- A common mistake is failing to *recognize futile intubation attempts* and failing to *move immediately to alternate/rescue airway interventions.* In general, limit emergency department (ED) attempts to three total laryngoscopies (regardless of number of operators). If initial laryngoscopy attempts are not successful, repeated attempts are unlikely to be successful and cause anatomic injury, increasing the difficulty of subsequent airway management efforts.
- *Have a low threshold for calling for help.* Often a second clinician can provide key input to help salvage the situation.
- Before performing laryngoscopy, *make sure that the patient can tolerate laryngoscopy.* Bradycardia or hypoxia may represent signs of impending cardiac arrest. The stress of laryngoscopy may increase the risk of cardiac arrest. It may be prudent to defer ETI attempts until the patient's physiology improves. Alternative strategies include continuing bag-valve-mask ventilation or inserting a supraglottic airway.

Basic Airway Interventions

Basic airway interventions are the cornerstone of airway and ventilatory support in the critically ill (see Table 15.1). *Nasal cannulae* provide low-flow (2–5 L/min) oxygen at inhaled fractions (FiO_2) ranging from 20% to 40%. Oxygen masks include *simple face masks* (6–10 L/min oxygen delivery, 40%–60% FiO_2) and *nonrebreather masks* (10–15 L/min oxygen delivery, close to 100% FiO_2). The latter contains a reservoir bag that must be fully inflated prior to patient application.

Patients with respiratory failure (apnea) or compromise should *receive bag-valve-mask ventilation (BVM)* (Fig. 15.1). At 10–15 L/min oxygen delivery, the BVM will deliver close to 100% FiO_2. To operate the BVM, the operator uses one hand (typically the left) to hold the mask to the face while simultaneously hyperextending the head to open the airway. The operator then uses the right hand to squeeze the ventilation bag. Because single-person BVM technique is difficult, use a two-person approach, with one operator using both hands to

Table 15.1 Airway Management Interventions

Basic airway interventions
Nasal cannula
Non-rebreather mask
Bag-valve-mask ventilation
Endotracheal intubation
Orotracheal intubation
Nasotracheal intubation
Other intubation techniques
Gum elastic bougie
Fiberoptic intubation
Video laryngoscopy tntubation
Supraglottic airways
Laryngeal Mask Airway (LMA™)
Esophageal Tracheal Combitube™ (ETC)
King Laryngeal Tube Airway (King LT™)
Surgical airways
Cricothyroidotomy
Transtracheal jet ventilation (TTJV)
Noninvasive positive pressure ventilation
Continuous positive airway pressure (CPAP)
Bilevel positive airway pressure (BiPAP)

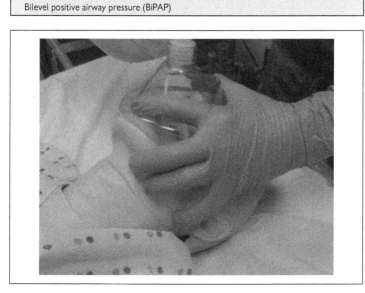

Figure 15.1 Bag-Valve-Mask Ventilation.

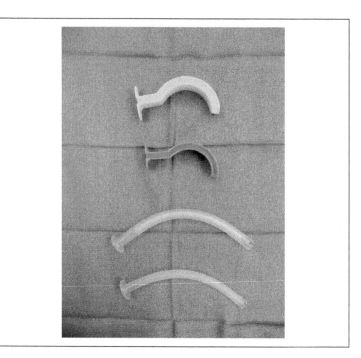

Figure 15.2 Oropharyngeal and Nasopharyngeal Airways.

hold and maintain mask seal and the other operator focusing on squeezing the self-inflating bag.[1]

The curved plastic *oropharyngeal airway* (Fig. 15.2) comes in several sizes and opens the airway by lifting the tongue forward from the posterior pharyngeal wall. Oropharyngeal airways should be reserved for patients without a gag reflex. A properly sized oropharyngeal airway should extend from the corner of the mouth to the angle of the mandible. The soft plastic *nasopharyngeal airway* lifts the soft palate and posterior tongue and may be used in any patient, including those with an intact gag reflex. A properly sized nasopharyngeal airway should extend from the corner of the mouth to the angle of the mandible. Practitioners should avoid inserting a nasopharyngeal airway in the presence of midface trauma; a fractured cribiform plate may result in inadvertent intracranial placement of the nasal airway.

Endotracheal Intubation

ETI is the standard method of advanced airway management in hospital settings, providing a direct conduit to the lungs to facilitate ventilation and isolate the airway from secretions and vomitus.

Orotracheal Intubation

This is the most common ETI method, using a lighted laryngoscope to expose the vocal cords for intratracheal placement of a plastic endotracheal tube (Fig. 15.3). Optimal orotracheal intubation requires the absence or near absence of airway reflexes; patients with intact protective airway reflexes usually require sedation and/or neuromuscular blockade (see section on "Rapid-Sequence Intubation").

Preparation is key to successful orotracheal intubation. The operator should place the patient supine and provide oxygenation by non-rebreather mask or a bag-valve-mask device. Have large-bore suction (e.g., Yankauer catheter) tested and ready at the bed and ensure that a well-functioning and proximal intravenous

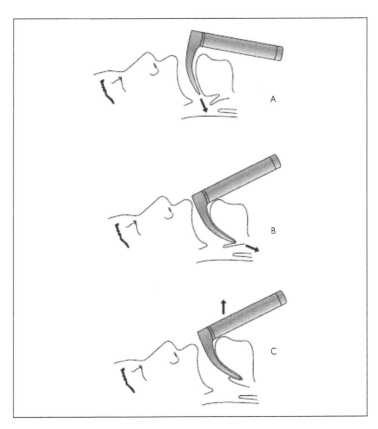

Figure 15.3 Standard orotracheal intubation technique.

(From Wang HE, Yealy DM. Airway Management. In Peitzman AB, Rhodes M, Schwab M, et al. (ed): The Trauma Manual: Trauma and Acute Care Surgery. Third edition. Lippincott, Williams and Wilkins, Philadelphia 2008).

line is present. (See "Rapid Sequence Intubation.") All patients should have continuous electrocardiographic, blood pressure cuff, and pulse-oximetry monitoring throughout care. In the absence of a suspected cervical spine injury, elevation of the head 2–4 cm with a small pillow ("sniffing position") may enhance atlanto-axial extension during laryngoscopy.[2] Some experts recommend that a second practitioner apply Sellick's or "BURP" maneuver, pushing backward on the cricoid membrane to prevent gastric insufflation and regurgitation[3]; we recommend these be done *selectively* rather than routinely since the benefits do not universally outweigh risks (impairing visualization or triggering vomiting).

A size 8.0–8.5 endotracheal tube is usually appropriate for an average-sized adult male, and a size 7.0–7.5 tube for an average sized adult female. Test each tube cuff by insufflating 10 mL of air before use. Some choose to insert a rigid, lightly lubricated stylet to aid handling and directing the ET tube.

The operator starts by inserting the laryngoscope into the right side of the patient's mouth and displacing ("sweeping") the tongue leftward. Contrary to popular belief, the laryngoscope does not directly elevate the tongue. The operator continues advancing the blade, exposing the epiglottis and glottic structures. The key anatomic structures are the epiglottis anteriorly/superiorly, the arytenoids posteriors/inferiorly, and the paired vocal cords extending between the epiglottis and arytenoids (Fig. 15.4).

The two most common laryngoscope blades—*Macintosh (curved)* and *Miller (straight)*—require different techniques (Fig. 15.5). With the curved Macintosh blade, the operator places the tip of the blade in the vallecula, pushing upon the hyoepiglottic ligament to indirectly elevate the epiglottis and expose the vocal cords. In contrast, the operator uses the broad side of the straight Miller blade to laterally displace the tongue, using the tip of the blade to *directly* lift the epiglottis.

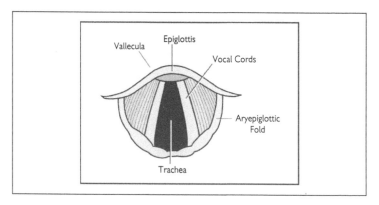

Figure 15.4 Laryngeal Structures.

(From Wang HE, Yealy DM. Airway Management. In Peitzman AB, Rhodes M, Schwab M, et al. (ed): The Trauma Manual: Trauma and Acute Care Surgery. Third edition. Lippincott, Williams and Wilkins, Philadelphia 2008).

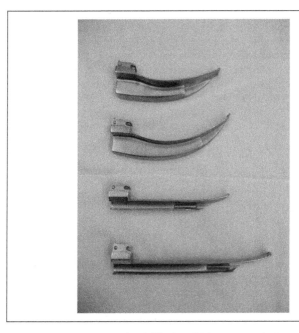

Figure 15.5 Macintosh (curved) and Miller (straight) Laryngoscope Blades.

Operators should limit the duration of each laryngoscopy attempt to 30 seconds—less if there is oxygen desaturation. Because each attempt creates additional airway trauma, limit to three total laryngoscopy attempts across all operators.

After exposure of the vocal cords, the operator places the endotracheal tube between the vocal cords and into the trachea. Using the markers on the side of the tube, the ET tube insertion *depth* should be approximately 22 cm at the patient's lip. The operator inflates the cuff with 10 mL of air and removes the stylet. The operator should confirm proper tube placement prior to securing the tube in place.

Nasotracheal Intubation

Nasotracheal intubation involves insertion of an endotracheal tube through the nose and into the trachea. Nasotracheal intubation is possible only on awake patients with intact respiratory efforts. While this approach is optimally used when the patient is awake, possesses intact protective airway reflexes, or when the patient cannot lay supine, it is rarely the ideal choice. Rapid sequence orotracheal intubation is often preferable.

The operator should choose an ET tube one-half size smaller than customary for orotracheal intubation. After liberally applying a water-soluble lubricant to the tube, the operator inserts the tube into the nares without a stylet, advancing the tube slowly toward the vocal cords. The right nares is typically larger and preferred. Fogging of the tube may be visible as the tube approaches the vocal cords. Some practitioners use a Beck Airway Advancement Monitor (BAAM) placed over the end of the endotracheal tube to guide insertion; the device whistles with each exhalation.[4] The operator coordinates endotracheal tube insertion through the vocal cords with patient inhalation. The Endotrol ET tube (Mallinckrodt Critical Care, St. Louis, Missouri) has a trigger that flexes the distal tip, aiding guidance of the tube through the vocal cords.

Other Intubation Techniques

The *Gum Elastic Bougie* is a semi-rigid stylet (Fig. 15.6). During laryngoscopy, the operator inserts the bougie through the vocal cords into the trachea. The bougie contains a rigid angled tip that provides tactile feedback as it rubs against the cartilaginous rings of the trachea. A conventional ET tube is inserted over the bougie and into the trachea.

Intubation with a *flexible fiberoptic bronchoscope* is difficult and requires specialized training. The operator first inserts the flexible fiberoptic bronchoscope through a standard endotracheal tube. He or she then guides the scope through the oropharnx, hypopharynx, and vocal cords, aiming to visualize the cartilaginous rings of the trachea. The endotracheal tube is then advanced over the scope into the trachea.

Video laryngoscopy uses a miniature digital video camera mounted at the tip of a specially designed laryngoscope blade, allowing the operator and others to

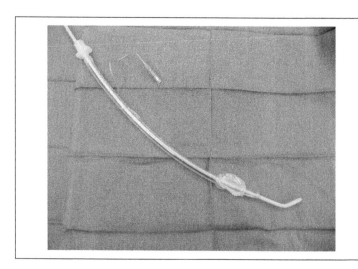

Figure 15.6 Gum Elastic Bougie.

view the glottic structures on a portable video monitor. These devices often allow indirect visualization of the vocal cords when direct visualization is limited or impossible. The most common video laryngoscopes currently used in the emergency department (ED) are the Glidescope (Verathon, Inc, Bothell, Washington) and Storz C-Mac (Tuttlingen, Germany). The operator may accomplish laryngoscopy and intubation using standard technique, either visualizing the vocal cord structure directly or indirectly with the video screen. Some video laryngoscope blades have an enhanced curve that requires the use of a specially designed stylet.

Confirmation of Endotracheal Tube Placement

Unrecognized misplacement of the endotracheal (ET) tube can rapidly result in hypoxia and death. *No single technique is adequate for confirming ET tube placement.* Because ET tube dislodgement may occur with movement of the patient, reconfirmation of ET tube placement should be performed whenever the patient is moved or transferred between stretchers.

While *auscultation* of the lungs and epigastrium is the most common method of tube placement confirmation, this approach is fallible. *End-tidal carbon dioxide detection* is the most accurate method for confirming proper ET tube placement. *Waveform end-tidal capnography* graphically display exhaled carbon dioxide waveforms, making it easier to interpret exhaled carbon dioxide patterns (Fig. 15.7). Waveform capnographers also allow for *continuous* verification of proper tube placement. *Digital end-tidal carbon dioxide capnometry* works on the same principle, except that the device displays peak carbon dioxide values rather than waveforms. *Colorimetric end-tidal carbon dioxide detectors* contain

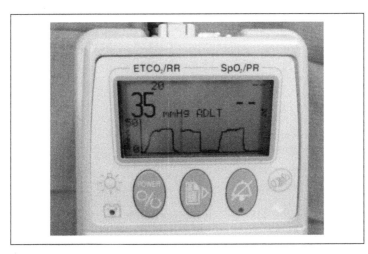

Figure 15.7 Waveform Capnography.

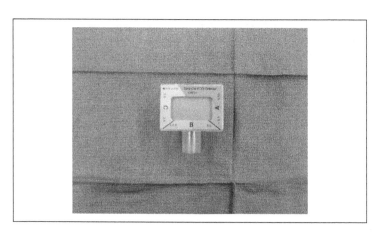

Figure 15.8 Colorimetric Carbon Dioxide Detector.

a chemically treated paper detector that changes color from purple to yellow when exposed to carbon dioxide (Fig. 15.8). Colorimetric carbon dioxide detectors are single use, have limited duration (<2 hours), and will not work if exposed to liquid.

While commonly performed after ETI, a chest X-ray is only useful for verifying correct ET tube depth, not tracheal placement. The presence or absence of ET tube fogging is an inaccurate indicator of ET tube position. Oxygen saturation is not a reliable indicator of tube placement since desaturation is often a late finding of misplacement. Direct revisualization of the ET tube placement is a viable technique for verifying tube placement but requires repeat laryngoscopy, which may not be possible if the tube has been secured in place.

Securing the Endotracheal Tube in Place

The ET tube must be secured to prevent inadvertent movement or dislodgement. The most common method is adhesive tape wrapped around the neck and the endotracheal tube (Lillehei method).[5] Many institutions use cloth umbilical "twill" tape to tie the tube in place. A variety of commercial tube holders also exist, incorporating a plastic bite-block strapped to the patient's face using Velcro tape, and a plastic strap or screw clamp to hold the endotracheal tube in place.

Ventilation after Intubation

During early phases after intubation, inadvertent hyperventilation is common and must be avoided. Hyperventilation has adverse effects upon cerebral blood flow in traumatic brain injury, coronary perfusion pressure during cardiopulmonary resuscitation, and cardiac output in hemorrhagic states.[6–8] Providers should aim for ventilation rate of no more than 12–15 breaths per minute, which corresponds to 4- to 5-second pauses between ventilations. The goal is normal or near-normal minute ventilation.

Intubation of the Trauma Patient

A salient concern in the trauma patient is the potential presence of a cervical spine fracture or injury. In these patients, a second rescuer must provide "manual in-line stabilization" of the cervical spine during orotracheal intubation to avoid risk of worsening any injury. Also, airway patency and laryngoscopy are achieved solely with lifting of the mandible, *without* hyperextension of the head or neck. Because of the potential for hypovolemia and traumatic brain injury, medications used to facilitate ETI must limit any reduction in blood pressure.

Intubation Adverse Events

Important adverse events to avoid during ETI efforts include the following:

- Unrecognized ET tube misplacement (esophageal or supraglottic)
- Endotracheal tube dislodgement
- Multiple laryngoscopy attempts
- Oxygen desaturation during laryngoscopy efforts
- Bradycardia during laryngoscopy efforts
- Airway injury
- Interruptions in CPR chest compressions during airway management. Some clinicians use supraglottic airways in this setting to avoid chest compression interruptions.

Supraglottic Airways

Inserted into the oropharynx, supraglottic airways allow ventilation without the use of an ET tube. Supraglottic airways provide a bridge intervention in the face of failed ETI or in place of perceived "likely to fail" ETI efforts. Some EMS practitioners use the King LT instead of the ETI as the primary airway in cardiac arrest because of the ease and performance. Most times after initial field and hospital care, clinicians will exchange a supraglottic airway with an ET tube (see section on "Converting a Supraglottic Airway to an Endotracheal Tube").

Laryngeal Mask Airway

The Laryngeal Mask Airway™ (LMA—LMA North America, San Diego, California) has a spade-shaped cuff that seals around the vocal cord structures (Fig. 15.9). The operator inserts the device blindly through the oropharynx, using the index finger to position the cuff around the laryngeal structures. Insufflation of the cuff with approximately 20–30 mL air facilitates a perilaryngeal seal. Practitioners should use estimated body weight to select the correct size adult LMA; 50–70 kg, size 4; 70–100 kg, size 5; >100 kg, size 6. The major complication of the LMA is aspiration. An LMA variant is the Intubating LMA (LMA™ "Fastrach"), specially designed to accommodate passage of an endotracheal tube later.

Esophageal Tracheal Combitube™

The Esophageal Tracheal Combitube™ (ETC or "Combitube"—Kendall Corporation, Kendall-Sheridan Catheter Corporation, Argyle, New York) is a

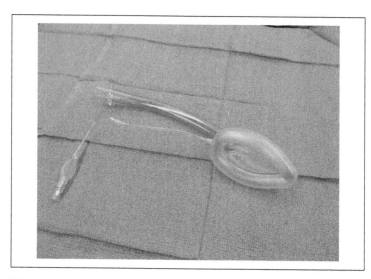

Figure 15.9 Laryngeal Mask Airway.

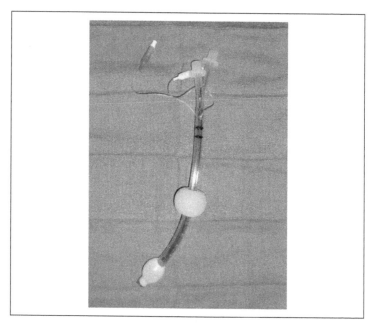

Figure 15.10 Esophageal-Tracheal Combitube.

double-lumen tube with distal and proximal balloons (Fig. 15.10). The operator inserts the Combitube blindly into the patient's mouth, positioning the smaller distal balloon in the esophagus and the larger proximal balloon in the oropharynx and inflating both cuffs. The operator first insufflates the taller blue tube; if the Combitube is properly placed, insufflated oxygen will exit fenestrations between the proximal and distal cuffs and enter the trachea, facilitating ventilation. If no ventilation occurs, the Combitube has been inserted in the trachea; the operator should switch ventilation to the shorter white port. Proper port selection may be assisted using end-tidal carbon dioxide detection. Complications associated with Combitube include choosing the wrong ventilation port, oropharyngeal bleeding, esophageal perforation, and aspiration pneumonitis. The standard Combitube is sized for patients >5' tall, while the Combitube SA is sized for individuals 4'–5'6" tall.

King Laryngeal Tube™

Popular in both prehospital and ED settings, the King Laryngeal Tube™ (King LT—King Systems, Noblesville, Indiana) airway appears similar to a Combitube but contains only a single lumen tube. Also, a single insufflation port inflates both proximal and distal balloon cuffs (Fig. 15.11). The King LT design is shorter than the

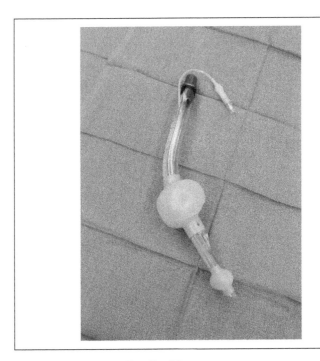

Figure 15.11 King Laryngeal Tube (King LT).

Combitube and facilitates more consistent placement in the esophagus. The complications of the King LT are similar to those reported for the Combitube, although the incidence of these events is not well studied. The technique of King LT insertion is similar to a Combitube. Appropriate adult sizes include the following: patient height 4–5 ft, size 3 (yellow); 5–6 ft, size 4 (red); and >6 ft, size 5 (purple).

Converting a Supraglottic Airway to an Endotracheal Tube

While supraglottic airways are suitable for temporary ventilation, ED clinicians may opt to convert the device to an endotracheal tube to reduce the risk of aspiration and limit mucosal damage from the supraglottic device cuffs. Options for converting a supraglottic airway to an ET tube include the following:

- *Remove the supraglottic device and perform conventional laryngoscopy.* While common, this is challenging if the supraglottic airway was initially inserted because of intubation difficulty. Operators should carefully assess the situation before proceeding with this option.

- *Convert the King LT airway blindly over a gum elastic bougie.* This is not possible with the Combitube or LMA. The operator inserts a gum elastic bougie blindly though the King LT into the trachea. The operator removes the King LT, leaving the bougie in place. The operator then passes a standard ET tube over the bougie. The pitfall of this technique is potential for inadvertent hypopharyngeal perforation.

- *Convert the LMA or King LT over a fiberoptic bronchoscope.* This technique is not possible with the Combitube. This technique requires the use of a special Aintree intubating catheter (Cook Medical, Inc., Bloomington, Indiana), which is similar to a bougie but is hollow, allowing insertion over a fiberoptic bronchoscope (Fig. 15.12). The operator places an Aintree catheter over the fiberoptic scope and guides the scope through the supraglottic airway, vocal cords, and into the trachea. The operator removes the fiberoptic scope and supraglottic airway, leaving the Aintree catheter in place. A standard ET tube may then be guided over the catheter into the trachea.

- *Leave the supraglottic airway in place and perform a cricothy- or tracheotomy.* Some clinicians favor this option when prior intubation efforts were difficult and/or the patient will likely require prolonged mechanical ventilation. While the ideal strategy is to bring the patient to the operating room for a controlled tracheostomy, placement of a surgical airway in the ED is possible.

A common misconception is that supraglottic airways must be immediately changed to an endotracheal tube. The appropriate technique and urgency for ET tube conversion depends upon the adequacy of ventilation through the supraglottic airway, the physiologic state of the patient, and the reasons for supraglottic airway insertion.

Surgical Airways

When attempts at ETI or supraglottic airway insertion have failed or are not possible (for example, severe facial trauma), the placement of a *surgical airway*

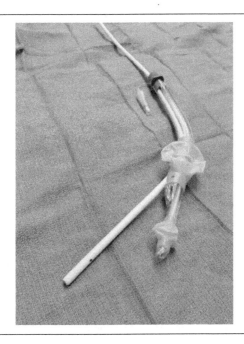

Figure 15.12 Exchanging a King LT over an Aintree catheter. The Aintree catheter is hollow, allowing insertion over a fiberoptic bronchoscope. Once guided into the trachea, the King LT may be removed, and an endotracheal tube may be inserted over the catheter into the trachea.

may be necessary. The key anatomic landmarks for surgical airway placement are the thyroid cartilage, the cricoid membrane, and the trachea (Fig. 15.13).

In a classic "open" *cricothyroidotomy* the operator stands to the patient's right side. Using the left hand, the operator locates and immobilizes the thyroid cartilage. Next, incise vertically from the middle of the thyroid cartilage to below the cricoid membrane with a #11 blade. After identifying the cricoid membrane (immediately inferior to the thyroid cartilage), the operator makes a horizontal 2-cm incision through the membrane. The operator then uses a tracheal hook to apply cephalad traction on the exposed membrane. A standard tracheostomy tube or small (size 6.0) ET tube is guided into the trachea. Pitfalls in open cricothyroidotomy include incision of the superior hypothyroid membrane instead of the inferior cricoid membrane, bleeding, or misplacement of the tracheal tube in the soft tissues rather than in the trachea. Commercial kits offer an alternate Seldinger-wire based approach to cricothyroidotomy (Fig. 15.14).

Transtracheal jet ventilation (TTJV) involves insufflation of high-pressured oxygen through a large-bore (>16-gauge) catheter inserted through the cricothyroid membrane. This technique requires a special oxygen regulator capable of

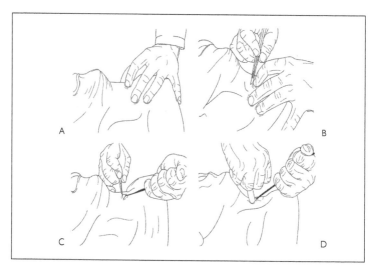

Figure 15.13 Open Cricothyroidotomy.

(From Brofeldt BT, Panacek EA, Richards JR. An easy cricothyroidotomy approach: the rapid four-step technique. Academic Emergency Medicine 1996:3:1060–1063).

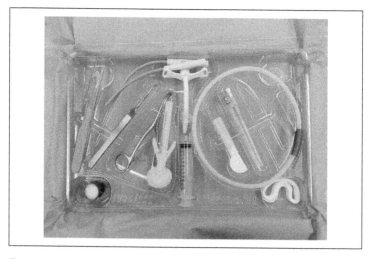

Figure 15.14 Mellker cricothyroidotomy kit. This kit facilitates cricothyroidotomy using Seldinger technique.

delivering oxygen at 40–50 L/min, available from *unregulated* tank or wall out-lets. TTJV cannot be performed using conventional bag valve mask equipment or a standard 25 L/min flow meter. TTJV is usually deployed for initial care, later either intubating under more controlled settings or converting the catheter site to an open cricothyroidotomy. Many clinicians mistakenly believe that TTJV facilitates oxygenation only rather than ventilation; a 16-gauge catheter with a flow rate >40–50 L/min and a ventilatory rate of 12–15/min will deliver normal or above-normal minute ventilation for prolonged periods (hours or even days).

Rapid Sequence Intubation and Other Drug-Faciliated Intubation Techniques

Orotracheal intubation is difficult or impossible in patients who are awake, combative or possess intact airway reflexes. Rapid sequence intubation (RSI) facilitates ETI through the use of a neuromuscular blocking (paralytic) agent combined with a sedative or induction agent. The goal of RSI is to gain rapid control of the airway and ventilation while minimizing unwanted hemodynamic effects (for example, blood pressure or intracerebral pressure increases). This application contrasts with the anesthesia term "rapid sequence induction," which denotes a strategy of rapidly achieving intubation while preventing regurgitation and aspiration of gastric contents.

   While some clinicians universally use RSI for all patients, the decision to use RSI or other drug agents should be made on an individual basis. The only absolute contraindication to RSI is a clinical scenario with anticipated unresolvable anatomic difficultly (e.g., jaw fracture, profound swelling, rigid neck, etc.) or an inability to mask ventilate a patient. Neuromuscular blockade ablates all protective airway reflexes and spontaneous respirations. If ETI or an alternate airway technique cannot be rapidly accomplished after pharmacologic paralysis, *the operator must stop and perform bag-valve mask ventilation* to avoid hypoxia and cardiac arrest. If the operator cannot safely perform RSI, he or she should select alternate options.

   RSI encompasses six major steps (the "6 P's"): (1) preparation, (2) preoxygenation, (3) pretreatment, (4) paralysis, (5) placement of ET tube, and (6) postintubation management.

Preparation

The patient should be positioned supine on the stretcher and have a secured intravenous line. Use continuous physiologic monitoring (electrocardiogram, blood pressure, and pulse oximetry) throughout and have large-bore suction immediately available. The operator should review relevant patient history for RSI drug contraindications, and he or she should assess airway anatomy and the anticipated level of difficulty. Also, have at least two rescue approaches—usually a supraglottic and surgical airway—immediately available at the bedside.

Preoxygenation

Preoxygenation of a healthy adult allows tolerance of up to 8 minutes of apnea prior to oxygen desaturation.[9] However, critically ill patients have impaired physiologic and pulmonary function plus lower oxygen reserves; even with extended preoxygenation, these individuals tolerate shorter periods of apnea prior to oxygen desaturation. The patient should receive oxygenation with a non-rebreather mask or bag-valve-mask ventilation until oxygen saturation is 100%, ideally for 3 minutes or more. Preoxygenation via BVM ventilation is less preferable, as it can result in inadvertent gastric insufflation, heightening the risk of regurgitation and aspiration.

Pretreatment

None of the pretreatments are recommended universally. *Lidocaine*, 1.5 mg/kg IV administered 3–5 minutes prior to laryngoscopy, may blunt heart rate, blood pressure, and intracerebral pressure increases from laryngoscopy, but the effect is tepid and is overcome by prolonged efforts. A small "defasciculating dose" of a nondepolarizing neuromuscular blocking agent (for example, *vecuronium* 1 mg IV) may attenuate the fasciculations of succinylcholine. The risk of this approach is that some will experience respiratory failure but not the flaccid paralysis needed for intubation. Because children often develop bradycardia in response to neuromuscular blocking agents, some clinicians give *atropine* (0.02 mg/kg, minimum 0.1 mg) to children prior to RSI.

Sedation and Paralysis

The goal is to rapidly create optimal and safe intubating conditions with patient comfort and lack of recall. Operators should give these drugs in rapid (over 3–5 seconds) consecutive boluses. The ideal RSI sedative/induction agent provides rapid and deep sedation, short duration, and minimal effects on blood pressure or intracerebral pressure. A prudent approach is to assume the presence of both hypovolemia and traumatic brain injury prior to intubation. Commonly used sedative/induction agents include the following:

- *Etomidate* (0.3 mg/kg IV; 20 mg in a 70 kg adult patient) is an imidazole-derived anesthesia induction agent. The onset of action is 30–60 seconds and duration action is <10 minutes. In trauma patients and many other critically ill patients, etomidate is favored because of reliable deep sedation and minimal blood pressure, heart rate, and intracranial pressure effects. However, etomidate may cause hypotension in select cases, particularly if severe hypovolemia is present. An important side effect of etomidate but with unclear clinical implications is adrenocortical suppression.[10] In a single dose, the clinical impact of this effect is uncertain but likely outweighed by the benefits.

- *Midazolam* (0.1 mg/kg; 7.0 mg in a 70-kg adult) is a short-acting benzodiazepine. Midazolam and other benzodiazepines may cause clinically significant hypotension.

- *Fentanyl* (2–5 μg/kg IV; 150–350 μg in a 70-kg adult) is an opioid with an onset of action of 1–2 minutes and a duration of action of 30–40 minutes. Fentanyl is less likely than other opioids to cause hypotension. Fentanyl can cause chest wall rigidity, but this is uncommon in these doses; treat this side effect with neuro-muscular blockade and intubation, which is usually planned in this setting.

- *Ketamine* (1–2 mg/kg IV; 70–140 mg in a 70-kg adult) is a dissociative anesthetic with onset of action in 30–60 seconds and duration of action for 5 minutes. Ketamine has few unwanted effects upon heart rate or blood pressure, making it an alternative in those with hypotension or severe volume depletion. It also may bronchodilate, making it attractive in severe asthmatic patients requiring intubation.Ketamine may raise intracranial pressure and should be used with caution in head injured patients.

- *Barbiturates* are used for RSI; for example, thiopental (3–5 mg/kg IV; 210–350 mg in a 70-kg adult) or methohexital (1–3 mg/kg; 70–210 mg in a 70-kg adult). Barbiturates have rapid onset (<1 minute) and short duration (thiopental—5–10 minutes; methohexital 4–6 minutes) but may cause profound hypotension and should be used with caution in acute resuscitation. We do not recommend barbiturate use outside of select setting (e.g., brain injury without hypovolemia or hypotension).

Long acting neuromuscular blocking agents are less desirable in the event of failed intubation efforts and the need to restore spontaneous patient respirations. Common RSI neuromuscular blocking agents include the following:

- *Succinylcholine* (1.0–2.0 mg/kg IV; 70–140 mg in a 70 kg adult) is the most commonly neuromuscular blocking agent used for RSI because of it fast, predictable onset (<1 minute) and short duration of action (5–7 minutes). A depolarizing agent, succinylcholine causes transient muscle fasciculations prior to onset of paralysis. The major side effect of succinylcholine is iatrogenic hyperkalemia, which may lead to cardiac arrest. Relative contraindications to succinylcholine use include conditions with known or potential hyperkalemia such as acute or chronic renal failure or rhabdomyolysis. Succinylcholine may be safely used for the initial management of burn and multiple trauma victims; hyperkalemia associated with these large body part injuries usually does not occur until 2 or 3 days after the acute injury. Other relative contraindications include patients with muscular wasting diseases or prolonged paralysis (leading to hyperkalemia), eye globe injuries, impending cerebral herniation, and pseudocholinesterase deficiency (succinylcholine use may cause prolonged neuromuscular blockade). Succinylcholine may raise intracranial pressure, but the clinical significance is likely absent in most patients—it is acceptable to use succinylcholine in the setting of traumatic brain injury.

- *Rocuronium* (0.6–1.2 mg/kg IV; 45–85 mg in a 70-kg adult) is a nondepolarizing agent with rapid onset (1–1.5 minutes) and moderate duration (20–30 minutes).

- *Vecuronium* (0.08–0.10 mg/kg IV; 5–7 mg in 70-kg adult) is a nondepolarizing agent with medium speed of onset (2–3 minutes) and long duration of action (30–35 minutes).[11] Some advocate higher doses (0.15–0.25 mg/kg IV; 11–18 mg in 70-kg adult) for faster onset of neuromuscular blockade. Rocuronium is likely a better choice for RSI than vecuronium due to its rapid onset and moderate duration.

Placement of Endotracheal Tube

Standard laryngoscopic technique may be used with RSI.

Postintubation Management

Verification of ET tube placement and securing of the ET tube should occur after intubation. (See earlier section on "Confirmation of Endotracheal Tube Placement.")

After intubation, the operator should give additional pharmacologic agents to maintain sedation. Intermittent doses of lorazepam (0.025–0.05 mg/kg IV; 2–4 mg in a 70-kg adult), midazolam (0.05–0.1 mg/kg; 3.5–7 mg in a 70-kg adult), diazepam (5–10 mg IV), or fentanyl (25–50 mcg IV) may be given. Propofol (5–50 mcg/kg/min continuous IV infusion, titrated to effect) may also be used if hypovolemia and hypotension are resolved.

If continued paralysis is required, longer acting neuromuscular blocking agents may be used. Vecuronium (initially 0.08–0.10 mg/kg IV; 5–7 mg in 70-kg adult) will provide 30–35 minutes of paralysis. Repeat lower doses of 0.01–0.02 mg/kg IV (2–4 mg in a 70-kg adult) will provide an additional 15–20 minutes of paralysis. The effects of neuromuscular blocking agents are cumulative—repetitive dosages may cause prolonged neuromuscular blockade.

Sedation-Only Intubation

Some promote giving a sedative agent only, without concurrent neuromuscular blockade, citing the preservation of native reflexes in the event of unsuccessful ETI efforts. However, this principle may not generalize to the ED, where patients are frequently too combative or awake; sedation alone may not create optimal intubating conditions. Also, some patients have compromised physiologic reserves and cannot tolerate the stress of laryngoscopy. The same concerns apply to the technique of topical anesthetic spray (benzocaine, etc.) assisted ETI.

Noninvasive Positive Pressure Ventilation

An important alternative to ETI, NIPPV delivers ventilatory support through a face or nasal mask, matching and augmenting the patient's spontaneous respiratory efforts. NIPPV may be useful for treating acute respiratory failure in patients with intact mental status and airway reflexes, potentially averting ETI. NIPPV reduces work of breathing, improves pulmonary compliance, and recruits atelectatic alveoli, keeping small airways open, increasing the available gas exchange area, and reducing ventilation-perfusion mismatch.[12] By increasing intrathoracic pressure, NIPPV increases hydrostatic pressure, shifting edema from the alveoli into the vascular system. The increased intrathoracic pressure also decreases cardiac venous return, transmural pressure, and afterload.

NIPPV is suitable for patients in acute respiratory distress but possessing intact ventilatory efforts, protective airway reflexes, and mental status. Patients with frank respiratory failure, apnea, absence of gag, or blunted mental status should receive ETI. While classically used to treat acute heart failure, some clinicians report success with other conditions such as pneumonia or asthma.

There are two types of NIPPV. *Continuous positive airway pressure (CPAP)* applies uniform supportive pressure during both inspiratory and expiratory phases. *Bilevel positive airway pressure (BiPAP)* is similar to CPAP but alternates different levels of inspiratory and expiratory pressure. CPAP may set to an initial level of 7 cm H_2O pressure support titrated up to 20 H_2O to clinical effect. In BiPAP systems the inspiratory and expiratory airway pressures are set separately; an inspiratory pressure of 10 cm H_2O with an expiratory pressure of 5 cm H_2O is a common initial setting, increasing support titrated to clinical effect.

Response to NIPPV should be assessed frequently through examination of work of breathing, respiratory rate, heart rate, blood respiratory, and oxygen saturation. Patients who fail to improve with NIPPV should receive ETI.

Mechanical Ventilator Management

This section highlights general principles of mechanical ventilator management to achieve these goals. The ultimate objectives of ED airway management are to ensure adequate oxygenation and ventilation.

Components of Mechanical Ventilation

Rate is the number of breaths per minute. While typical settings range from 12 to 30 breaths/minute, the optimum ventilatory rate depends upon the clinical scenario. While increased rates may be preferable in select patients (for example, those with acute lung injury), hyperventilation (and resulting high minute ventilation) may be harmful in traumatic brain injury, cardiac arrest, or hypotension.

Tidal volume (TV) is the volume of each delivered breath and is usually based upon the patient's body weight. While widely used in clinical practice, *conventional TV* (10–15 ml/kg) may cause alveolar overdistension during inspiration and collapse during expiration, causing acute lung injury. Studies suggest reduced mortality and fewer complications with *low TV* (6–8 mL/kg).[13] *Minute ventilation* (rate x tidal volume) is the total volume of ventilation delivered in 1 minute.

Fraction of inspired oxygen (FiO₂) refers to the percentage of oxygen in each delivered breath and may range from 40% to 100%. Prolonged hyperoxia can cause increased free radical production, leading to cellular damage and increased mortality.[14] Thus, as soon as possible after intubation, FiO₂ should be titrated downward to maintain an arterial oxygen saturation of approximately 90%.

By limiting full exhalation, *positive end-expiratory pressure (PEEP)* creates elevated expiratory pressure to keep alveoli open, improving gas exchange, increasing lung compliance, and increasing PaO2. PEEP may prove helpful in the presence of lung pathology such as pneumonia or acute lung injury.

Compliance refers to the ability of the proximal and distal airways to distend. Conditions such as acute lung injury (ALI) limit lung compliance, increasing the airway pressures necessary to inflate proximal and distal airways. Because distal airways are more sensitive to increased pressures, conditions that decrease compliance heighten the risk of lung injuries. Examples of conditions that decrease compliance include acute respiratory distress syndrome, pneumonia, pulmonary edema, air-trapping/auto-PEEP, pneumothorax, and atelectasis.

Resistance refers to the ability of the proximal airway to respond to changes in pressure. In patients with conditions that increase resistance (asthma, chronic obstructive pulmonary disease [COPD]), increased inspiratory pressure may be required to inflate the proximal and distal airways.

Peak airway pressure refers to the maximal air pressure at the end of inspiration. Normal peak airway pressures range from 15 to 30 cm H_2O. Clinicians should maintain peak airway pressures below 30 cm H_2O to avoid barotrauma. Increased resistance or decreased compliance can result in increased peak pressures. Isolated elevated peak pressures indicate increased resistance, for example, from mucus plugs or bronchospasm.

Plateau airway pressure refers to the airway pressure after inspiration but before expiration. Normal plateau airway pressures are below 30–35 mm H_2O. The plateau pressure is directly related to the compliance of the lung. The difference between peak (resistance and compliance) and plateau airway pressures (compliance) is the airway resistance. Elevation of both peak and plateau airway pressures indicates decreased compliance.

Inspiratory:expiratory (I:E) ratio refers to the respective duration of the inspiration and expiration phases. The typical I:E ratio is 1:2 with an inspiratory flow rate of 60 L/min. Alteration of the I:E ratio may be required in select situations. For example, the bronchospasm associated with asthma and COPD may require a prolonged expiratory phase.

Modes of Mechanical Ventilation

In *volume-cycled ventilation*, the delivered volume is fixed while the pressure is allowed to vary. In *pressure-cycled ventilation*, the delivered pressure is fixed while the volume is allowed to vary. Because uncontrolled tidal volumes (>10 mL/kg) can result in lung injury, volume-cycled ventilation is the preferred ventilation strategy.

Assist-control ventilation (AC) is the standard method of ventilation and delivers breaths at fixed tidal volumes and rate. AC mode may also be set with additional delivered breaths whenever the patient initiates extra breaths over the set rate. AC ventilation delivers a set tidal volume with each breath, potentially leading to stacking of breaths, increased intrathoracic pressure, barotrauma, decreased venous return, and hypotension (Fig. 15.15).

Pressure support ventilation (PSV) delivers breaths of set inspiratory pressure synchronized with the patient's spontaneous breathing efforts without a set tidal volume or respiratory rate. PSV may be used in patients with spontaneous respiratory efforts and is often used for "weaning" from mechanical ventilation.

Synchronized intermittent mandatory ventilation (SIMV) is similar to AC ventilation but allows the patient to breathe at an independent rate and tidal volume between mandatory breaths. The utility of SIMV remains controversial.

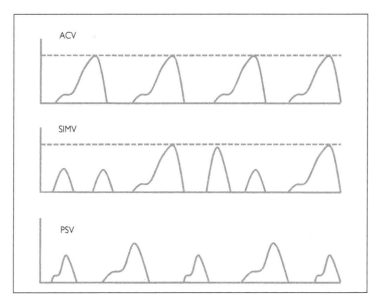

Figure 15.15 Mechanical ventilator modes. ACV, Assist Control Ventilation; SIMV, Simultaneous Intermittent Mandatory Ventilation; PSV, Pressure Support Ventilation

Although breath stacking and auto-PEEP are more common in AC, they may also occur with SIMV. Breath stacking and auto-PEEP are more pronounced in individuals with left-ventricular dysfunction; therefore, AC is preferred over SIMV in this population.

Adjustment of Ventilator Parameters

Adjustment of ventilation parameters is guided by information from arterial blood gas results ($PaCO_2$ and PaO_2) or exhaled end-tidal carbon dioxide ($ETCO_2$) levels. In very general terms, target normal levels are $ETCO_2$ and $PaCO_2$ = 40 mm Hg, and PaO_2 = 75–100 mm Hg. If the $PaCO_2$ or $ETCO_2$ is too high, raise the respiratory rate; conversely, if the $PaCO_2$ or $ETCO_2$ is too low, lower the respiratory rate. If the ABG PaO_2 is too low, raise FiO_2, tidal volume, respiratory rate, or PEEP. If the ABG PaO_2 is too high, lower FiO_2, tidal volume, respiratory rate, or PEEP. *High concentration oxygen is toxic.* Lower FiO_2 to 50% or lower as soon as possible after intubation. These are very general guidelines; specific management also depends upon the physiologic state of the patient and the selected ventilator mode.

Complications of Mechanical Ventilation

ED clinicians must look for and be prepared to manage a range of common ventilator complications. Aspiration may occur because the seal of the ET tube cuff is not adequate to completely prevent entry of oral secretions and gastric contents into the airway. Frequent suctioning and elevation of the head of the bed (to between 30 and 45 degrees) may help to mitigate aspiration. *Tracheal tube cuff underinflation* may impair ventilation and increase the risk of aspiration, while an *overinflated cuff* can damage the surrounding tracheal tissue, leading to tracheal necrosis. ET tube cuffs should be inflated to 20–25 mm Hg. *Tracheal tube dislodgement* may occur even with a properly secure tube.

Mucous plugs can occlude the airway, leading to atelectasis and impairing oxygenation. Treatment consists of direct suctioning, aerosolized or instilled N-acetylcysteine, or bronchoscopy. *Pneumothorax* may occur in up to 15% of ventilated patients. *Reduced cardiac output* may occur with mechanical ventilation from increases in intrathoracic pressure and excessive minute ventilation, which may impair venous return and preload, resulting in decreased cardiac output.

ALI is characterized by diffuse endothelial and epithelial lung tissue injury, resulting in decreased lung compliance, hypoxemia, and pulmonary edema. Strategies to prevent ALI include the use low tidal volumes (6–8 mL/kg), limiting plateau airway pressures (<30 cm H_2O), and limiting respiratory rate to <30 breaths/minute.[13]

Pearls of Care

1. *Preparation is key.* This includes best possible positioning, oxygenation, and verification of proper working equipment.
2. *Anticipate the difficult airway.* All emergent airways should be considered difficult.
3. *Plan ahead.* The initial plan plus second and third choices should be clear and ready before starting.
4. *Do not wait for desaturation or catastrophe to use a rescue/alternate airway.* It is acceptable to defer intubation efforts and proceed directly to supraglottic or surgical airway insertion.
5. *Avoid hyperventilation.* Controlled ventilation requires discipline and monitoring.

References

1. Davidovic L, LaCovey D, Pitetti RD. Comparison of 1- versus 2-person bag-valve-mask techniques for manikin ventilation of infants and children. *Ann Emerg Med* 2005;46:37–42.

2. Greenland KB, Eley V, Edwards MJ, Allen P, Irwin MG. The origins of the sniffing position and the Three Axes Alignment Theory for direct laryngoscopy. *Anaesth Intensive Care* 2008;36(Suppl 1):23–27.

3. Baskett PJ, Baskett TF. Resuscitation great. Brian Sellick, cricoid pressure and the Sellick Manoeuvre. *Resuscitation* 2004;61:5–7.

4. Cook RT, Jr., Stene JK, Jr . The BAAM and endotrol endotracheal tube for blind oral intubation. Beck Airway Air Flow Monitor. *J Clin Anesth* 1993;5:431–432.

5. Carlson J, Mayrose J, Krause R, Jehle D. Extubation force: tape versus endotracheal tube holders. *Ann Emerg Med* 2007;50:686–691.

6. Davis DP, Dunford JV, Poste JC, et al. The impact of hypoxia and hyperventilation on outcome after paramedic rapid sequence intubation of severely head-injured patients. *J Trauma* 2004;57:1–8; discussion -10.

7. Aufderheide TP, Lurie KG. Death by hyperventilation: a common and life-threatening problem during cardiopulmonary resuscitation. *Crit Care Med* 2004;32:S345–S351.

8. Pepe PE, Lurie KG, Wigginton JG, Raedler C, Idris AH. Detrimental hemodynamic effects of assisted ventilation in hemorrhagic states. *Crit Care Med* 2004;32:S414–S420.

9. Benumof JL, Dagg R, Benumof R. Critical hemoglobin desaturation will occur before return to an unparalyzed state following 1 mg/kg intravenous succinylcholine. *Anesthesiology* 1997;87:979–982.

10. Zed PJ, Mabasa VH, Slavik RS, Abu-Laban RB. Etomidate for rapid sequence intubation in the emergency department: is adrenal suppression a concern? *CJEM* 2006;8:347–350.

11. Walls RM. Rapid-sequence intubation in head trauma. *Ann Emerg Med* 1993;22:1008–1013.

12. Hillberg RE, Johnson DC. Noninvasive ventilation. *N Engl J Med* 1997;337:1746–1752.

13. Amato MB, Barbas CS, Medeiros DM, et al. Effect of a protective-ventilation strategy on mortality in the acute respiratory distress syndrome. *N Engl J Med* 1998;338:347–354.

14. Kilgannon JH, Jones AE, Shapiro NI, et al. Association between arterial hyperoxia following resuscitation from cardiac arrest and in-hospital mortality. *JAMA* 2010;303:2165–2171.

Chapter 16

Ultrasound for Shock

Robert J. Hyde

Introduction

Emergency ultrasonographic examination of the patient with shock offers a rapid and noninvasive approach to diagnostic and therapeutic decision making. Although not intended to replace comprehensive ultrasonographic examinations by others, point-of-care emergency and critical care ultrasound has benefits that have the potential for improving patient outcomes. The concept of bringing ultrasound technology to the patient is highlighted in this instance, whereby clinicians contemporaneously perform and interpret ultrasonographic imaging. Maintaining an awareness of the patient's clinical milieu while gathering diagnostic data permits dynamic patient management and the ability to intervene rapidly. The increased availability, portability, and adoption of ultrasound technology into clinical practice among emergency and critical care providers also permit the dynamic reassessment of an evolving clinical course. Data derived from an ultrasonographic examination can help redirect clinicians to ascertain the cause for hypotension and the shock state, thereby avoiding cognitive traps and errors.

Focused, goal-directed examinations that seek to answer a set of clinical questions in a timely fashion are key. As rapidly performed, limited evaluative tools, bedside ultrasound protocols visualize many abnormal physiologic states but do not exclude the presence of a pathologic state. Alternative imaging modalities, further evaluation, and specialty consultation may be required to exclude a given condition.

Key areas to evaluate in shock, which are amenable to ultrasonographic analysis, include the following:

The heart, including hemodynamics
The vasculature: aorta, deep venous system
The potential spaces: pericardium, peritoneum, pleural space

Additional areas may also be appropriately investigated and may provide useful diagnostic information as warranted by the patient scenario and clinical acumen.

The Heart and the Role of Echocardiography—Targets

1. Is the heart beating? At first glance, the question seems somewhat absurd, one that should be easily answerable without the use of ultrasound. However, low-flow or no-flow states can be difficult to clinically evaluate, especially when patients are unresponsive and/or attached to a ventilator. Ultrasound is useful in differentiating reversible causes of pulseless electrical activity—severe hypovolemia, cardiac tamponade, massive pulmonary embolism, and tension pneumothorax. The ultrasonographic evaluation of each of these conditions is discussed separately later. Establishing ventricular activity may alter management decisions; for example, the management strategy for the patient with ventricular tachycardia without a pulse differs from the patient who has demonstrated evidence of cardiac output. When there is complete absence of cardiac motion and a sonographic diagnosis of cardiac standstill is made, current resuscitative efforts may not be effective.

   a. Acquiring a subcostal four-chamber view of the heart is recommended for this purpose. The subcostal view is routinely obtained in the supine patient, and if chest compressions are anticipated or in progress, the subcostal probe position will not interfere with hand placement on the sternum for compressions.

2. Is the heart beating effectively? Gross ventricular function can be quickly assessed at the bedside. Global assessment of contractility can be visually estimated or calculated using numerous methods and/or formulas. Evaluation of left ventricular (LV) size and contractility is useful in determining whether cardiogenic shock is present or if other conditions exist. A semi-quantitative visual estimation is adequate for guiding initial resuscitative efforts, especially when time is a factor and a major concern. One commonly used scheme is to classify LV function as either hyperdynamic, normal, impaired, or severely impaired. M-mode can assist with this analysis. LV function is typically assessed in the subcostal, parasternal, and apical windows. Clinical status may prevent patient repositioning, but when feasible, elevating the left arm over the head and/or moving the patient into a left lateral decubitus position serves to open the intercostal spaces, brings the heart closer to the chest wall, and improves overall image acquisition.

3. Is there a pericardial effusion? Rapid identification of fluid around the heart is an important step that should be taken early to determine whether cardiac tamponade is responsible for the shock state. Although only a minority of patients with pericardial effusion will have tamponade physiology, seeing more than trace pericardial effusion in the critically ill patient may be assumed to be a causative factor of hypotension until confirmatory imaging and/or pericardiocentesis is performed. In the parasternal long axis view, a key landmark to identify is the descending thoracic aorta (DTA). Pericardial fluid will be seen as an anechoic collection anterior to the DTA. Pleural effusion, which may also be present and confound the

evaluation, is seen tracking posterior to the DTA. Most patients with cardiac tamponade will have associated moderate to large effusions, but small rapidly accumulating effusions may also cause hemodynamically significant changes in the intrapericardial pressure gradient. Pericardial effusion with right atrial diastolic collapse is a highly sensitive echocardiographic finding for cardiac tamponade and is best seen in the apical or subcostal four-chamber views. Early echocardiographic findings for cardiac tamponade include increased respiratory variation in transvalvular flow velocities (tricuspid valve followed by mitral valve.) In the hemodynamically unstable patient who requires pericardiocentesis, ultrasound helps identify the shortest distance from the skin surface to the effusion and the location of its maximum size. By optimizing the conditions where the pericardiocentesis needle is inserted and directed, echocardiography enhances the success rate and limits complications compared to traditional methods. The identification of pericardial fluid can also suggest alternate diagnoses. For example, pericardial effusion seen together with an enlarged aortic root in a patient complaining of chest pain should prompt consideration of aortic dissection.

a. Large, circumferential effusions are detectable in any single window, but smaller and/or loculated effusions may be more difficult to detect if only one view is obtained. It is best to survey the pericardial space in multiple views to confirm the presence and extent of pericardial effusion rather than to rely on a single view for this purpose. In so doing, mimics such as pericardial fat pads and ascitic fluid can be more readily distinguished from pericardial effusion.

4. Is there right ventricular (RV) strain? RV dysfunction is a common finding in critically ill patients and may be related to an acute, chronic, or acute-on-chronic etiology. The assessment of RV size in comparison to the LV is a straightforward, rapid, objective, and practical means of detecting RV dilation. This may be accomplished in parasternal long axis window, but many sonologists prefer to image and compare the ventricles in the apical or subcostal four-chamber view. The RV:LV ratio should be less than 0.6. When the RV:LV ratio >1, severe dilation exists.

a. RV strain is not a diagnosis; instead, its presence alerts the provider to a number of possible scenarios, including chronic obstructive pulmonary disease, obstructive sleep apnea, pulmonary hypertension, pulmonary embolism, RV infarction, and acute left heart failure creating secondary right heart strain. In the hemodynamically unstable patient, RV strain may be the result of massive pulmonary embolism and the causative agent for obstructive shock, prompting consideration of fibrinolytic therapy.

b. The absence of RV enlargement and dysfunction should not be used to exclude the diagnosis of pulmonary embolism. Visualization of thrombus within the right heart or pulmonary artery is an infrequent finding but prompts the need for aggressive treatment and/or surgical consultation in the unstable patient. Other indirect echocardiographic findings of acute pulmonary embolism include hypokinesis of the RV free wall sparing the apex (McConnell's sign), a D-shaped left ventricle in the parasternal short axis view, abnormal interventricular septal motion, and a plethoric IVC. Evaluation of the deep venous system should also be undertaken in the appropriate clinical context when pulmonary embolism is suspected, and this is discussed separately later.

5. Is an acute valvular disorder suspected requiring surgical intervention? Although extensive training in echocardiography is recommended to study valve structure and function comprehensively, a limited examination can aid when evaluating the patient in shock. For example, acute and catastrophic mitral and/or aortic valve dysfunction should be considered in the hemodynamically unstable patient, and these disorders should prompt surgical consultation and comprehensive echocardiographic evaluation when suspected.

   a. Limited two-dimensional TTE findings that should raise concern for severe valve failure include abnormal valve architecture, noncoaptation or prolapse of the valve leaflets, and/or the presence of an oscillating intracardiac mass on a valve or adjacent structure. For example, a prominent flail leaflet may be identified in the parasternal long axis view and is usually associated with severe MR. The addition of color Doppler, spectral Doppler, two-dimensional imaging or transesophageal echo adds additional diagnostic information.

6. Is the patient intravascularly replete? Assessment of the inferior vena cava (IVC) can be rapidly performed at the bedside to estimate central venous pressure and intravascular volume status. It is frequently assessed during the echocardiographic examination using the same transducer.

   a. The IVC is relatively compliant and is expected to collapse during inspiration due to the expansion of the thoracic cavity, generation of negative intrapleural pressure, and increased venous return. IVC diameter measurements can be assessed throughout the respiratory cycle and used as a surrogate to differentiate right atrial pressures and intravascular volume status. Low right atrial pressure (<5 mm Hg) is associated with a small-diameter IVC (<1.5 cm) and significant respiratory collapse (>50%). IVC dilation (>2.5 cm) without significant respiratory collapse (<50%) indicates a high right atrial pressure (>15 mm Hg). Due to physiologic changes that occur during positive pressure ventilation, these parameters may not be reliable in the mechanically ventilated patient. However, even in this subset of patients, a small-diameter or collapsed IVC reliably excludes elevated right atrial pressures.

   b. IVC evaluation should be interpreted in the clinical context. A small-diameter IVC in the setting of a hypercontractile, small left ventricle is consistent with the hypovolemic state and fluid therapy is appropriate. Similarly, the decision to withhold fluid administration in favor of inotropic or afterload reduction therapy in the patient with a hypocontractile left ventricle and pulmonary edema seems straightforward.

c. IVC size alone does not necessarily predict the need for fluid therapy. The patient who presents with septic shock, for example, may demonstrate echocardiographic evidence of impaired contractility and have variable IVC measurements. The decision to administer fluids, and if so, how much fluid to administer before adding vasopressors becomes a more complex choice. When a strategy of fluid administration is chosen, serial IVC measurements can be useful as a means of determining fluid responsiveness following volume administration and may signal the need for vasopressor support (i.e., when the IVC exhibits dynamic changes, <50% respiratory variability or exceeds a minimum caliber).

d. IVC size does not predict fluid responsiveness. Many providers will empirically administer fluid challenges to hypotensive patients presumed to be in shock, while attempting not to induce fluid overload resulting in pulmonary edema and respiratory failure. Lung sonography may aid, particularly if B-lines (the sonographic equivalent of pulmonary edema) are detected during the course of fluid resuscitation. The B-line is an air-fluid artifact that correlates with pulmonary edema and may be present in any interstitial disease. However, following aggressive fluid resuscitation in shock, B-lines most likely represent resultant hydrostatic edema. B-lines are frequently detectable before fluid overload is clinically apparent.

The Vasculature—Targets

1. Is an abdominal aortic aneurysm (AAA) present? A minority of AAA cases presenting to the ED will have the classic clinical features of back pain, a pulsatile abdominal mass, and hypotension. Sonographic detection of AAA is confirmed when the diameter of the aorta exceeds 3 cm or when there is a 50% increase in the diameter of the aorta compared to the uninvolved proximal segment. The aorta should be scanned in both the sagittal and transverse plane, from the diaphragm to the iliac bifurcation. Measurements should be taken in the transverse (short-axis) plane from outer wall to outer wall. Be careful to avoid underestimating the diameter of the vessel, especially when heterogeneous, echogenic-appearing, thrombotic debris has accumulated in between the outer wall of the aorta and the true lumen. Such findings can be subtle but must be included when calculating the vessel diameter. When abnormal findings and sonographic evidence for AAA is visualized in the hypotensive patient, immediately consult a surgeon for repair.

2. Is an aortic dissection present? Thoracic aortic dissection, like AAA, can present subtlyand without classic features such as severe back pain ("tearing"), hypertension and pulse asymmetry, and neurologic dysfunction.

The sonographic sign of aortic dissection is the intimal flap, seen as a linear, mobile echogenic stripe separating the true lumen from the false lumen of the vessel. The echogenic flap appears within the anechoic lumen. In the appropriate clinical context, the presence of a widened aortic root (>4 cm) with concurrent pericardial effusion may also suggest the diagnosis. If this aotic root change is seen, act quickly, as impending cardiac tamponade is common. When the intimal flap of aortic dissection propagates in a retrograde direction and involves the origin of a coronary artery, significant regional wall abnormalities may be present. Correlation with electrocardiogram findings may be helpful and is recommended. Severe AR may also develop, although astute clinicians will recognize that both AR and regional wall abnormalities may represent preexisting cardiac disease. Once dissection is detected, consult a surgeon immediately.

3. Is deep venous thrombosis (DVT) present? Since most pulmonary emboli originate from the lower extremities, looking for DVT is helpful in unstable patients or those with chest pain, dyspnea, or hypotension. Compression ultrasonography provides a simple, accurate, and rapid means to evaluate for DVT. Using a high-frequency linear transducer, the vein of interest is examined in its short axis and gentle downward pressure is applied with the probe. Failure of the vein to completely collapse indicates the presence of thrombosis. The common femoral vein, at its junction with the greater saphenous vein, should be interrogated for this purpose. The probe is swept distally to permit inspection and compression of the deep femoral and superficial femoral veins. The probe is then picked up and the leg is placed in a dependent position to promote maximum venous capacitance. In the popliteal fossa, the popliteal vein is examined down to its trifurcation in the calf, using the same compression technique and analysis.

   a. Upper-extremity venous thrombosis can be assessed using the same compression technique if clinically indicated or suspected. When preparing for venous access and selecting a target vessel, ultrasonographic evaluation of the vein to test for the presence of thrombus is recommended prior to needle insertion.

The Potential Spaces—Focused Exams

1. The extended focused assessment with sonography in trauma (eFAST) was developed to evaluate the trauma patient. Positive findings predict the need for operative management. The views that are obtained during the eFAST exam can aid care of patients who present with hypotension absent trauma. Since the heart and the pericardial space have already been discussed previously, attention is now given to the hepatorenal interface, the perisplenic and splenorenal interface, the rectovesicular/rectouterine spaces, and the pleural space.

a. Sonographically detectable free fluid may represent blood, ascites, urine, pleural effusion, contents from a ruptured viscous and/or other abnormal fluid collection. Differentiating blood from other fluids may not be possible based upon history alone. Blood may have a heterogeneous, echogenic appearance depending upon whether the clot has had time to develop. In the actively bleeding patient, fresh blood appears echogenic, but as clot develops, echo texture is frequently seen. Sampling is often necessary for definitive diagnosis.

2. Is there free fluid in the chest or abdomen? In the abdomen, free fluid accumulates in the most dependent portions of the body. In the supine hypotensive patient, the hepatorenal interface or Morrison's pouch is the most dependent region. To ease free fluid identification, reposition the patient either head down or feet down if circumstances allow. Be sure to scan the entire interface of adjacent organs (i.e., liver and kidney) so as not to miss key pathologic findings. Move the probe over the skin surface until the organ(s) of interest is visualized coming into view and then going out of view. It is the apposition of these structures that defines the potential space, and the sonologist must be vigilant when performing the examination.

   a. In the hypotensive childbearing age woman, test for pregnancy. If positive and free fluid is noted in the abdomen or pelvis, ectopic pregnancy is suspected – consult an obstetrician. In cases involving third-trimester pregnancy, position patients the lateral decubitus position to prevent the gravid uterus from compressing the IVC.

3. Is there free fluid in the chest? In the chest, evaluate both hemithoraces for hemothorax and/or effusion. In the axillary region, the key landmark to identify is the diaphragm, seen as an echogenic curved line, to differentiate free fluid in the chest from the peritoneum. Loss of mirroring artifact suggests the presence of free fluid in the abdomen. A subtle and indirect finding in the presence of thoracic free fluid is the extension of the spinal stripe beyond the diaphragm. When identified, further thoracic evaluation is prudent to identify relevant pathology.

   a. Ultrasound permits rapid, accurate diagnosis of pneumothorax, particularly in the supine patient. This rapid detection aids whenever intubation and positive pressure ventilation are used or considered. With the transducer held steady and perpendicular to the skin in a longitudinal plane, the pleural line is visualized between adjacent ribs and assessed dynamically. Lung sliding, which represents the movement of the pleural surfaces against each other during ventilation, excludes the diagnosis of pneumothorax. Comet tail artifact or lung rockets, seen as vertical echogenic lines, are also seen in normal lung and absent with pneumothorax. When there is ambiguity with the diagnosis, compare with the contralateral chest.

Pearls of Care

1. Bedside, point-of-care ultrasound requires training and practice.
2. Always merge the image results with the clinical picture to optimize decisions.
3. Make sure you do not exclude options with focused US exam (aside from cardiac activity)—it is best used to guide care when direct findings are seen.
4. Visualize all of the organs you are assessing—partial views equate to missed findings.
5. Store your images for care documentation and to improve.

Selected Readings

Beaulieu Y. Bedside echocardiography in the assessment of the critically ill. *Crit Care Med* 2007;35:S235–S249.

Blaivas M, Fox JC. Outcome in cardiac arrest patients found to have cardiac standstill on bedside emergency department echocardiogram. *Acad Emerg Med* 2001;8:616–621.

Labovitz AJ, Noble VE, Bierig M, et al. Focused cardiac ultrasound in the emergent setting: a consensus statement of the American Society of Echocardiography and American College of Emergency Physicians. *J Am Soc Echocardiogr* 2010;23:1225–1230.

Levitov A, Mayo P, Slonim A. *Critical Care Ultrasonography.* New York: McGraw-Hill; 2009.

Lichenstein DA. *Whole Body Ultrasonography in the Critically Ill.* Berlin: Springer-Verlag; 2010.

Meredith EL, Masani ND. Echocardiography in the emergency assessment of acute aortic syndromes. *Eur J Echocardiogr* 2009;10:i31–i39.

Perera P, Mailhot T, Riley D, Mandavia De. The RUSH exam: rapid ultrasound in shock in the evaluation of the critically ill. *Emerg Med Clin N Am* 2010;28:29–56.

Royse CF. Ultrasound-guided haemodynamic state assessment. *Best Pract Res Clin Anaesthesiol* 2009;23:273–283.

Tsung T, Enriquez-Sarano M, Freeman WK, et al. Consecutive 1127 therapeutic echocardiographically guided pericardiocenteses: clinical profile, practice patterns and outcomes spanning 21 years. *Mayo Clin Proc* 2002;77:429–436.

Volpicelli G. Usefulness of emergency ultrasound in nontraumatic cardiac arrest. *Am J Emerg Med* 2011;29:216–223.

Zoghbi WA, Enriquez-Sarano M, Foster E, et al. Recommendations for evaluation of the severity of native valvular regurgitation with two-dimensional and doppler echocardiography. *J Am Soc Echocardiogr* 2003;16:777–802.

Chapter 17

Blood Product and Procoagulant Use

Edward P. Sloan and Donald M. Yealy

Introduction

Blood transfusion in the emergency department usually occurs in one of three settings: (1) in patients with massive hemorrhage, (2) in patients with chronic anemia in whom even modest additional blood loss causes physiological dysfunction, and (3) in patients with abnormal hemostasis due to disrupted clotting factor or platelet functioning. Procoagulants help attenuate bleeding, especially (but not limited to) that caused or worsened by anticoagulants.

The transfusion of packed red blood cells (PRBCs) may improve oxygen carrying capacity and cellular oxygenation in the setting of hemorrhage and shock. Component transfusion is given to augment hemostasis by replacing blood components such as plasma, platelets, and clotting factors. Procoagulant therapies such as prothrombin complex concentrates (PCCs) or recombinant factor VIIa (rFVIIa) additionally enhance clotting cascade functioning in the setting of hemorrhage or disrupted hemostasis as a result of therapeutic anticoagulation. Hemoglobin-based oxygen carriers (HBOCs) are in development for use in the setting of acute hemorrhagic shock when blood is not available.

Specific blood or procoagulant uses are discussed in other sections of the text; this chapter reviews the general principles, highlighting a few key deployments.

Definition of Terms

Whole blood transfusion provides all of the components of blood, including RBCs, white blood cells, platelets, clotting factors, and plasma. Historically, donor whole blood was mixed with an anticoagulant and was transfused after cross-matching without the need for other processing. However, current blood banking practice involves separation of donated blood into one or more of its RBC, plasma, cryoprecipitate, and platelet components.

Packed red cell (PRBC) units have a hematocrit of up to 65%, a volume of 250 to 310 mL, and can be stored at 1°C–6°C for up to 42 days. During storage, drops in RBC 2,3-DPG levels cause a left shift in the oxygen dissociation curve and impaired RBC oxygen delivery to the periphery so that the transfused RBCs less effectively improve tissue oxygenation. Shortly after each PRBC unit is transfused, the measured hemoglobin (Hb) will rise by about 1 g/dL, and the hematocrit will rise by 3%–4%. PRBC transfusion may cause rigors from the noncellular content or trigger transfusion associated lung injury (TRALI, an ARDS-like event), the latter usually with larger transfusion volumes. With today's blood handling procedures, true PRBC mismatch-related reactions are exceptionally rare and usually from human error during sampling, labeling, or delivery.

Fresh frozen plasma (FFP) is frozen at −18°C or less within 8 hours of collection from the donor. It can be used for up to 1 year from freezing after being thawed at 37°C. A unit of FFP from one donor unit of blood contains about 250 mL of plasma, proteins, and nonconcentrated clotting factors. A typical 10–15 mL/kg FFP transfusion of 3–5 units, with a volume of 750–1250 mL, will provide factors II, V, VII, IX, X, and XI. TRALI can occur after large-volume FFP transfusion.

Platelets are pooled from up to 10 donors or via platelet apheresis from a single donor. While both sources provide effective platelets for transfusion, the single-donor method allows for a reduced number of donor exposures, making it the theoretically safer method of platelet transfusion. Each unit of whole blood–derived platelets contains up to 1×10^{11} platelets, and each apheresis-derived unit can contain up to six times that number of platelets. As such, the typical platelet transfusion is six or more units of whole blood–derived platelets or one unit of single-donor, apheresis-derived platelets. This will result in an increase in the platelet count of approximately 30,000/mL when measured 1 hour after the transfusion. Platelet transfusion in those with intracranial bleeding during antiplatelet drug use is discussed in Chapter 9; in general, platelet transfusions solely for this indication lack strong evidence of benefit. TRALI remains a potential after large-volume platelet therapy.

Cryoprecipitate is obtained from thawed and centrifuged FFP and contains factor VIII, fibrinogen, fibronectin, factor XIII, and von Willebrand factor (vWF). Although this low-volume clotting factor concentrate can be used to restore fibrinogen levels or to treat hemophilia, other therapies such as recombinant factors are the preferred method for restoring these clotting proteins.

Prothrombin complex concentrate (PCC) solutions are procoagulants derived from plasma. In the United States, PCCs contain factors II, IX, and X. In Canada and the European Union, PCCs contain factors II, VII, IX, X, and proteins C and S. In patients with acute hemorrhage or when there are diminished clotting factor levels due to liver disease or warfarin anticoagulation, these products can be dosed based on the initial international normalized ratio (INR) and patient body mass to normalize the INR within minutes of infusion.

Recombinant factor VIIa (rFVIIa) is a protein that exerts a hemostatic effect interaction with tissue factor in the presence of vascular injury. Although it is approved by the Food and Drug Administration only for use in hemophilia patients, it is also given in a body mass–based dose in those with acute injury and blood loss.

Table 17.1 Transfusion Protocol for Hemorrhagic Shock Patients

- Assess for the signs of class III hemorrhage and uncompensated or partially compensated shock, then rapidly infuse crystalloids (not colloids).

- Do not use large volumes of crystalloid *alone* when blood loss is severe or ongoing. *Start PRBC early* and infuse multiple PRBC units simultaneously.

- In acute large-volume blood loss, use type O, Rh-negative PRBC units in women of childbearing age and type O, Rh-positive PRBC units in everyone else.

- In ongoing/uncontrolled hemorrhage, allow for permissive hypotension (targeting 90 mm Hg systolic blood pressure) during volume resuscitation to minimize blood losses and coagulopathy—restoring normal pressure after bleeding is controlled.

- In symptomatic patients with blood loss, immediately send a blood sample to the blood bank for type and cross matching.

- Inform the blood bank of the need for the rapid delivery of cross-matched PRBC units and the possible need for a massive transfusion whenever type O blood is transfused.

- Outside of shock/ongoing blood loss, transfuse cross-matched PRBCs units one at a time if feasible to seek any possible transfusion reactions.

- Consider early emergency department–initiated TXA in the trauma patient with symptomatic hemorrhage.

- Continually assess signs for critical end-organ dysfunction, acute lung injury, and the laboratory abnormalities that include Hb/Hct, coagulation profile, calcium, and lactic acid in those receiving massive transfusions.

Hemoglobin-based oxygen carriers (HBOCs) are solutions with oxygen-carrying capacity that mimic the use of blood in the management of acute blood loss and hemorrhagic shock, especially in out-of-hospital settings where blood is not immediately available. None are currently approved for human use in the United States.

Tranexemic acid (TXA) is a non-blood-based procoagulant that inhibits plasmin and plasminogen activity. While available for decades, it is gaining popularity in the care of those with trauma-related hemorrhage.

Vitamin K is used to reverse warfarin coagulopathy, though reversal can take hours. *Protamine sulfate* can reverse heparin coaguloapathy.

Clinical Syndromes and Pathophysiology

Acute Hemorrhagic Shock

In the setting of acute hemorrhagic shock, lost intravascular blood volume is first replaced with infusions of crystalloid and blood products (Table 17.1). In the initial resuscitation of hemorrhagic shock patients, colloids such as albumin or FFP do not improve outcomes compared to crystalloids and are not utilized.

Acute trauma resuscitation practice currently utilizes permissive hypotension to a target systolic blood pressure of 90 +/− 10 mm Hg rather than seeking "normal blood pressure." This allows reduced total volume of fluid and blood products infused, which may reduce the frequency of coagulopathy and lung complications in trauma patients. The utilization of blood salvage techniques in the emergency department and operating room in patients with massive hemorrhage may also assist in decreasing the total volume of allogeneic blood transfused.

PRBCs are transfused immediately for hemorrhagic shock patients who have lost 30% (or 1500 mL) of an estimated 5000 mL total blood volume and/or patients with ongoing blood loss and signs of uncompensated shock. For emergent needs, use type O, Rh-negative blood in women of childbearing ages and type O, Rh-positive blood in men and all other women. In one large series, no acute hemolytic transfusion reactions were seen with this approach and only 1 of 10 who received a large volume of type O, Rh-positive blood developed antibodies to the Rh antigen.

Following the transfusion of type O blood or when time permits, use cross-matched PRBC and other blood component therapies if needed. Ideally, cross-matched blood can be delivered in about 30 minutes, limiting the need for the transfusion of type-specific blood. In the absence of severe hemorrhagic shock, single PRBC units should be transfused serially to best assess the etiology of possible transfusion reactions.

An important issue in the setting of uncontrolled or profoundly symptomatic hemorrhage is the *transfusion ratio* of PRBCs to other blood components. The American Association of Blood Banks defines massive transfusion as 10 or more PRBC units per day, with a recommended FFP to PRBC ratio >1:3. FFP infusion during the acute resuscitation of hemorrhagic shock patients may improve trauma mortality and morbidity. Data from 11 retrospective studies of component to PRBC ratios, including massive hemorrhage patients, suggest that a ratio of FFP to PRBC units >1:2 provides a survival benefit. In submassive transfusion for trauma patients, a transfusion ratio >1:1 FFP to PRBC had nearly a two-fold greater survival, improved coagulation parameters, and decreased blood product use up to 48 hours. Similarly, an increased platelet to PRBC ratio of >1:2 is associated with increased survival at 24 hours and 30 days.

When considering the ratios of all three of these blood component therapies, the total PRBC volume transfused is the most critical determinant of these blood transfusion ratios. In a study of severely injured trauma patients who were transfused with greater than 10 PRBC units, a PRBC:FFP:platelet ratio of 1:1:1 increased survival and decreased complications. However, a similar review of 1788 US trauma patients transfused with less than 10 PRBC units in the first 24 hours, those transfused with FFP:PRBC and platelet:PRBC ratios >1:2 had greater morbidity as measured by greater ventilator and intensive care unit days, without any improvement in mortality. As such, it may be important to limit the use of FFP and platelet transfusions to those patients who are actively bleeding and in whom six or more PRBC units have been transfused.

In acute traumatic hemorrhage, civilian and military trials show reduced mortality when TXA is given in the first hours. The effect on specific bleeding sites (e.g., intracranial hemorrhage) is less clear and induced thrombotic events do not appear more prevalent. TXA is not approved yet for this indication but is gaining popularity and is inexpensive. The role in other types of large-volume acute bleeding, notably gastrointestinal hemorrhage, is also not defined. The TXA dose is 1 g over 10 minutes IV followed by another 1 g over the next 8 hours.

Physiologic Derangement in Chronic Anemia Patients

In patients with chronic anemia who become critically ill or injured, the most important question is whether a more aggressive Hb transfusion trigger of 10 g/dL is superior to a lower Hb trigger of 7 g/dL. A review of 45 studies found that the benefits of PRBC transfusion outweighed the risks in only one study and one subgroup of patients, those with acute myocardial infarction and a hematocrit less than 30%. Additionally, PRBC transfusion was associated with greater odds of mortality (1.7x), infection (1.8x), and ARDS (2.5x). In a Cochrane Collaboration review, a transfusion trigger of 7 g/dL reduced exposure to blood by about one-third and reduced infection rates by one-quarter, making it a reasonable trigger given no clear patient benefit from the more aggressive blood transfusion Hb trigger of 10 g/dL.

Although most chronic anemia patients do not suffer clinically significant symptoms until their Hb falls below 7 g/dL, patients with heart or lung disease may become symptomatic and require transfusion when their Hb drops below 10 g/dL. An Hb transfusion threshold of 10 g/dL is utilized in early goal-directed therapy for patients with severe sepsis and a central venous saturation <70%. The clinical utility of this aspect of sepsis management, which has been questioned, is detailed further in Chapter 2.

In children, a restrictive transfusion trigger Hb level of 7–9 g/dL is appropriate, with a more liberal trigger being appropriate in preterm infants, in children with cyanotic heart disease, or in the settings of severe hypoxemia, active bleeding, or hemodynamic instability.

Blood Product Use in Patients with Abnormal Hemostasis

Patients may have abnormal hemostasis either due to therapeutic anticoagulation or antiplatelet drug use, or when there is clotting factor or platelet dysfunction.

The most common scenario is caring for a patient on warfarin therapy. For patients without active bleeding and an INR <5, no reversal is needed; temporary cessation of warfarin is best. If the INR is >5, deliver vitamin K (5–10 mg either orally or by slow IV to avoid hypotension). Add other procoagulants (FFP or PCC) when clinical bleeding or rapid reversal for interventions is desired.

Other newer oral anticlotting agents such as dabigatran and rivaroxaban have no reversal agents; some advocate using PCC if available for rivaroxaban or emergent dialysis for dabigatran-associated hemorrhage if bleeding site control fails, but neither is well studied.

In the rare setting where heparin must be reversed because of clinically important bleeding or an impending intervention, give 1 mg protamine sulfate IV for every 100 units of active heparin. Protamine can also reverse enoxaparin, albeit less effectively.

Although PCC solutions can reverse vitamin K antagonist anticoagulation within minutes, they are not yet widely available in the United States. Optimal PCC dosing occurs by including initial INR, target INR, and patient body mass in the dose calculation. In one study, thrombotic events occurred in 1.5% of 460 patients who received PCCs for rapid anticoagulation reversal.

FFP is more commonly used to quickly correct clotting deficiencies outside platelet-based maladies; it is rarely associated with thrombotic complications, it takes longer than PCC to administer, may cause fluid overload, and is associated with TRALI. A European review of coagulation factor concentrates (including PCC) in trauma patients demonstrated comparable mortality outcome in patients treated with PCC or FFP, with less short-term blood product use and lower organ failure complication rates with the former.

rFVIIa is extensively studied in patients with trauma and hemorrhage but has not yet been approved for this clinical use. In two studies, those who received rFVIIa had improved odds of 24-hour survival but not the longer term in-hospital survival. In the United States military, rFVIIa use over a 5-year period was not associated with an improvement in outcome or an increase in complications as compared to those who received standard therapy. For patients with intracerebral hemorrhage, adult cardiac surgery, and torso trauma, there was no survival benefit with rFVIIa use as compared to standard therapy, although for the torso trauma patients there was a reduced ARDS risk. The Cochrane Collaboration found no patient benefit with the potential for increased thromboembolic events. rFVIIa use has neither been shown to prevent intracranial hemorrhage in traumatic brain injury patients, nor has it been shown to improve outcomes in patients with spontaneous intracerebral hemorrhage.

Multiple studies of thrombocytopenic intensive care unit patients demonstrated a poor platelet transfusion response, defined as an increase of less than 30×10^9 per L after receiving six pooled platelet units. While often ordered when the platelet count is below 20,000 (esp. if below 10,000), data neither support prophylactic platelet infusions nor the use of a specific platelet count at which platelets should be infused in patients with marrow failure causing the thrombobyctopenia. Platelets are often given prior to an invasive procedure when the count is less than 50,000, again absent strong evidence. In children, platelets should not be infused in patients with TTP or heparin-induced thrombocytopenia unless a life-threatening hemorrhage has occurred. *Transfusion of platelets solely to correct antiplatelet drug effects* is currently unsupported by outcome data.

Hemoglobin-Based Oxygen Carrier Use

Hemoglobin-based oxygen carriers (HBOCs) are red blood cell–free solutions that are able to deliver oxygen to the periphery. Although many solutions have been developed, none have been demonstrated to improve outcome as compared to standard hemorrhage resuscitation that includes PRBC transfusion. The successful development of a clinically useful HBOC in humans will require that the solution be safe and at least as effective as PRBCs when used in the treatment of hemorrhagic shock patients. It will also need to be able to be safely stored at room temperature, allowing its use in out-of-hospital settings, including the military field, where blood is not immediately available for transfusion

Pearls of Care

1. Use balanced ratios of PRBCs, FFP, and platelets when transfusing six or more PRBC units in hemorrhagic shock patients.
2. In severe hemorrhagic shock, immediately transfuse type O blood, using type-O Rh-negative units for women of childbearing age.
3. Any trauma patient who receives blood in the emergency department is at a higher risk of meeting massive transfusion thresholds in the next 24 hours; notify the blood bank when using even one unit PRBC initially to allow preparation.
4. For most chronic or subacutely anemic patients, a transfusion trigger of 7 g/dL is appropriate. When end-organ dysfunction exists, especially cardiac ischemia, use a transfusion trigger of 10 g/dL.
5. Treat patients with critical illness or injury and a coagulopathy with bleeding with a transfusion of FFP and/or platelets. Procoagulant therapy with PCCs and rFVIIa may soon be added tools.
6. Avoid platelet transfusions for prophylaxis or to correct antiplatelet drug effects.

Acknowledgments

The author would like to thank James Clark for his assistance in searching the medical literature and Patricia Lee, MD, for her review of this chapter.

Selected Readings

Brown LM, Aro SO, Cohen MJ, Trauma Outcomes Group. A high fresh frozen plasma: packed red blood cell transfusion ratio decreases mortality in all massively transfused trauma patients regardless of admission international normalized ratio. *J Trauma* 2011;71(2 Suppl 3):S358–S363.

Carless PA, Henry DA, Carson JL, Hebert PP, McClelland B, Ker K. Transfusion thresholds and other strategies for guiding allogeneic red blood cell transfusion. *Cochrane Database Syst Rev* 2010;10:CD002042.

Curry N, Hopewell S, Dorée C, Hyde C, Brohi K, Stanworth S. The acute management of trauma hemorrhage: a systematic review of randomized controlled trials. *Crit Care* 2011;15(2):R92.

Holcomb JB, Zarzabal LA, Michalek JE, et al. Increased platelet: RBC ratios are associated with improved survival after massive transfusion. *J Trauma* 2011;71(2 Suppl 3):S318–S328.

Iorio A, Marchesini E, Marcucci M, Stobart K, Chan AK. Clotting factor concentrates given to prevent bleeding and bleeding-related complications in people with hemophilia A or B. *Cochrane Database Syst Rev* 2011;9:CD003429.

Lin Y, Stanworth S, Birchall J, Doree C, Hyde C. Recombinant factor VIIa for the prevention and treatment of bleeding in patients without haemophilia. *Cochrane Database Syst Rev* 2011;(2):CD005011.

Napolitano LM, Kurek S, Luchette FA, et al. Clinical practice guideline: red blood cell transfusion in adult trauma and critical care. *Crit Care Med* 2009;37(12):3124–3157.

Perel P, Roberts I, Shakur H, Thinkhamrop B, Phuenpathom N, Yutthakasemsunt S. Haemostatic drugs for traumatic brain injury. *Cochrane Database Syst Rev* 2010;1:CD007877.

Roberts I, Shakur H, Ker K, Coats T, on behalf of the CRASH-2 Trial collaborators. Antifibrinolytic drugs for acute traumatic injury. *Cochrane Database Syst Rev* 2011;1:CD004896.

Yank V, Tuohy CV, Logan AC, et al. Systematic review: benefits and harms of in-hospital use of recombinant factor VIIa for off-label indications. *Ann Intern Med* 2011;154(8):529–540.

Index